HEALTH LITERACY
AMONG OLDER ADULTS

Karen Kopera-Frye, PhD, Biedenharn Endowed Chair and Professor in Gerontology, Department Chair, Director of ULM's Institute of Gerontology, University of Louisiana at Monroe. Dr. Kopera-Frye received her BA, MA, and PhD from Wayne State University, Detroit, MI, in Developmental and Clinical Psychology/Gerontology, Department of Psychology and graduate Aging certification from there. She completed a Postdoctoral Fellowship at the University of Washington, Department of Psychiatry and Behavioral Sciences. She has conducted research on elder issues for 27 years including older adult health promotion. Dr. Kopera-Frye came to the University of Louisiana at Monroe as the Endowed Chair in Gerontology/Professor from the University of Nevada-Reno in Fall 2009. She became interested in health literacy in 2007, when she was selected for specialized training as a Scholar in Health Literacy through a grant awarded to the University of Nevada-Reno's Geriatric Education Center. Her research interests include health literacy, health promotion in older adults (e.g., successful aging), working with ethnically diverse elders, intergenerational projects, custodial grandparents, elderly inmates in prisons, and alcohol abuse among older adults. Dr. Kopera-Frye has been extensively involved in grantsmanship, and has been trained federally as an evaluator by Substance Abuse and Mental Health Services Administration (SAMHSA) and served as reviewer for the National Science Foundation. She is very active in the Gerontological Society of America (GSA) and the Association for Gerontology in Higher Education (AGHE). She received AGHE's Distinguished Teacher Award for her outstanding teaching utilizing service learning pedagogy and was awarded Fellow status. As a member and Fellow of GSA's Behavioral Social Science Section, she has been involved in GSA and AGHE governance activities including being appointed to the AGHE Task Force on Accreditation of Gerontology, an invited presenter at the AGHE Pre-Conference Teaching Institute, and a member of the AGHE Academic Program Development Committee. She has published extensively and serves as reviewer for journals such as *The Gerontologist*. She has served as a Member at Large on American Psychological Association's Division 20: Division on Adult Development and Aging (APA D20) most recently. Dr. Kopera-Frye noticed an absence of textbooks available to train our future professionals in health literacy among elders; hence, the idea for this textbook was born.

HEALTH LITERACY AMONG OLDER ADULTS

Karen Kopera-Frye, PhD
EDITOR

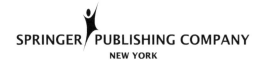

SPRINGER PUBLISHING COMPANY
NEW YORK

Springer Publishing Company, LLC
11 West 42nd Street
New York, NY 10036
www.springerpub.com

Acquisitions Editor: Sheri W. Sussman
Compositor: diacriTech

ISBN: 978-0-8261-9451-0
e-book ISBN: 978-0-8261-9452-7

Instructor's Materials: Qualified instructors may request supplements by emailing textbook@ springerpub.com:
Instructor's PowerPoints: 9780826121677

16 17 18 19 20 / 5 4 3 2 1

The author and the publisher of this Work have made every effort to use sources believed to be reliable to provide information that is accurate and compatible with the standards generally accepted at the time of publication. The author and publisher shall not be liable for any special, consequential, or exemplary damages resulting, in whole or in part, from the readers' use of, or reliance on, the information contained in this book. The publisher has no responsibility for the persistence or accuracy of URLs for external or third-party Internet websites referred to in this publication and does not guarantee that any content on such websites is, or will remain, accurate or appropriate.

Library of Congress Cataloging-in-Publication Data

Names: Kopera-Frye, Karen, editor.
Title: Health literacy among older adults / Karen Kopera-Frye, PhD, editor.
Description: New York, NY : Springer Publishing Company, LLC, [2017] |
   Includes bibliographical references and index.
Identifiers: LCCN 2016024068| ISBN 9780826194510 | ISBN 9780826194527 (ebook)
Subjects: LCSH: Health literacy. | Older people—Health and hygiene.
Classification: LCC RA773.74 .H418 2017 | DDC 613/.0438—dc23 LC record available at
https://lccn.loc.gov/2016024068

Special discounts on bulk quantities of our books are available to corporations, professional associations, pharmaceutical companies, health care organizations, and other qualifying groups. If you are interested in a custom book, including chapters from more than one of our titles, we can provide that service as well.

For details, please contact:
Special Sales Department, Springer Publishing Company, LLC
11 West 42nd Street, 15th Floor, New York, New York 10036-8002
Phone: 877-687-7476 or 212-431-4370; Fax: 212-941-7842
E-mail: sales@springerpub.com

Printed in the United States of America by McNaughton & Gunn.

Contents

Contributors

J. Scott Brown, PhD
Associate Professor
Department of Sociology & Gerontology
Miami University
Oxford, Ohio

Patti T. Calk, OTD, MEd, LOTR
Associate Professor and Associate Director of the School of Health Professions
Master of Occupational Therapy Program
University of Louisiana at Monroe
Monroe, Louisiana

Cathleen Carney-Thomas, DHSc, MA, CCP-SLP
Assistant Professor, Communication Sciences and Disorders
Indiana State University
Terre Haute, Indiana

Tommie Church, PhD
Assistant Professor of Kinesiology in School of Health Professions
University of Louisiana at Monroe
Monroe, Louisiana

Donna Eichhorn, MEd, LOTR
Assistant Professor
Master of Occupational Therapy Program
University of Louisiana at Monroe
Monroe, Louisiana

Iris Feinberg, PhD
Assistant Director, Adult Literacy Research Center
Georgia State University
Atlanta, Georgia

Daphne Greenberg, PhD
Distinguished University Professor of Educational Psychology, Special
Education, and Communication Disorders
Adult Literacy Research Center, College of Education & Human Development
Georgia State University
Atlanta, Georgia

Ronald A. Harris, PhD
Associate Professor of Public Administration in the School of Management
University of San Francisco
San Francisco, California

Jane G. Keehan, PhD, PT, OCS
Clinical Assistant Professor of Doctor of Therapy Program
Cleveland State University
Cleveland, Ohio

Kerry S. Kleyman, PhD
Assistant Professor of Psychology
Metropolitan State University
St. Paul, Minnesota

Karen Kopera-Frye, PhD
Biedenharn Endowed Chair
Professor in Gerontology
Director, Institute of Gerontology,
University of Louisiana at Monroe
Monroe, Loiusiana

Darren Liu, DrPH
Assistant Professor
Department of Health Care Administration and Policy
University of Nevada–Las Vegas
Las Vegas, Nevada

Erick B. López, MA
Doctoral Student
Department of Sociology
University of Nevada–Las Vegas
Las Vegas, Nevada

Tara P. McCoy, MA
Doctoral Student
Social/Personality Program, Department of Psychology
University of California–Riverside
Riverside, California

Julie McKinney, MS
Health Literacy Consultant
Health Literacy Consulting, Inc.
Cambridge, Massachusetts

Lori M. Metzger, PhD, CRNP
Assistant Professor
Diploma, Presbyterian University of Pennsylvania School of Nursing
Bloomsburg University of Pennsylvania, Nursing Department
Bloomsburg, Pennsylvania

Jennifer Michael, MSRS, RT(R)
Assistant Professor
School of Allied Health
Northwestern State University
Bossier City, Louisiana

Mary K. Milidonis, PhD, PT
Associate Professor, Physical Therapy Program
College of Sciences and Health Professions
Cleveland State University
Cleveland, Ohio

Carolyn Murphy, OTD, MA, LOTR
Associate Professor
Master of Occupational Therapy Program
University of Louisiana at Monroe
Monroe, Louisiana

R. V. Rikard, PhD
Postdoctoral Research Associate, Social Scientist
Department of Media and Information
Michigan State University
East Lansing, Michigan

Tracy A. Riley, PhD, RN, CNS, CNE
Professor
Mount Carmel College of Nursing
Columbus, Ohio

Samer N. Roy, MD
Internal Medicine
West Monroe, Louisiana

Denny G. Ryman, EdD, MT
Dean of Health Sciences
Theresa Patnode Santmann School of Health and Sciences
State University of New York, Farmingdale State College
Farmingdale, New York

Shreya Sahay Saxena, MD
Physician
Smolensk State Medical Academy
Smolensk, Russia

Krishnakant Shah (aka Khandelwal), MD
Physician
Smolensk State Medical Academy
Smolensk, Russia

Theresa B. Skaar, MA
Doctoral Student
Interdisciplinary PhD Program in Social Psychology
University of Nevada–Reno
Reno, Nevada

Anthony A. Sterns, PhD
CEO, iRxReminder LLC
Senior Lecturer and Fellow
Institute for Life-Span Development and Gerontology
The University of Akron
Akron, Ohio

Adjunct Professor
The University of Maryland University College
Adelphi, Maryland

Jennifer M. Stevens, MA
Doctoral Student in Sociology
Department of Sociology
University of Nevada–Las Vegas
Las Vegas, Nevada

Alexandra Talbott-Welch, SPT, BA
Doctoral Student in Physical Therapy
Cleveland State University
Cleveland, Ohio

Amani Talwar, MS
Doctoral Student in Educational Psychology
College of Education and Human Development, Dean's
Doctoral Research Fellow
Georgia State University
Atlanta, Georgia

Takashi Yamashita, PhD
Assistant Professor
Department of Sociology
University of Nevada–Las Vegas
Las Vegas, Nevada

Preface

Health literacy is the degree to which individuals have the capacity to obtain, process, and understand basic health information and services needed to make appropriate health decisions (Ratzan & Parker, 2000). More than one-third of all American adults, or 89 million individuals, lack sufficient health literacy to effectively understand and complete needed medical treatments and participate in preventive health care. Inadequate health literacy is more commonly noted in certain demographic groups such as the older adults, the poor, ethnically diverse groups, people with limited education, and people who did not speak English during early childhood. Only 12% of adults have proficient health literacy, according to the National Assessment of Adult Literacy (NAAL). In other words, nearly nine out of 10 adults may lack the skills needed to manage their health and prevent disease. These adults were more likely to report their health as poor (42%) and are more likely to lack health insurance (28%) than adults with proficient health literacy (Kirsch, Jungeblut, Jenkins, & Kolstad, 1993).

Low health literacy has been shown to correspond with greater hospitalization rates and use of emergency services, and use of services to treat disease rather than to prevent it (Scott, Gazmararian, Williams, & Baker, 2002)—all of which result in higher health care costs (Howard, Gazmararian, & Parker, 2005). It is such an important issue that it has been a priority area in *Healthy People* initiatives since 2010 and continues to be a priority area in current initiatives. What is particularly startling is the low level of health literacy among elders. The NAAL indicated the following about older adults' health literacy skills: 71% of adults aged 60+ years had difficulty in using print materials; 80% had difficulty using documents such as forms or charts; and 68% had difficulty with interpreting numbers and doing calculations. Older adults use more medical services and acquire more chronic illnesses than other population segments. By 2030, 71.5 million adults aged 65+ years will be living in the United States. This demographic shift and the NAAL data affirm that improving health information and services is a priority in any effort to achieve improved health for older adults (CDC, 2011). When patients cannot understand the diagnosis, treatment regimen, or prescription medication directions, it is a recipe for deleterious outcomes for those patients.

To address the intertwined problems of low health literacy and health disparities, the American Medical Association and others have recommended that health care professionals use plain language and visual aids, focus on the most important part of a health message, and use the teach-back method, in which clinicians explicitly request that patients repeat instructions using their own words (Weiss, 2007). Health professionals have been using various strategies to improve understanding of health-related information.

The purpose of this book is to provide a tool for training our future professionals in working with elders as clients, patients, and loved ones. There is no other textbook that specifically tackles this very important health care issue. The intent is for this book to be used in teaching graduate students, whether as a primary or supplemental textbook. Contributors include leaders in the field from across a broad array of professional disciplines. Thus, this textbook can be used in a stand-alone Health Literacy course or in a discipline-specific course such as nursing. The point is that health literacy cuts across all fields, and this text is suitable for training future occupational therapists as well as public health scientists. The character of this text is truly interprofessional, yet all contributors know that increasing health literacy is a key issue in their fields. Therefore, no matter what type of client a student may face on the job, health literacy will be involved. Though particularly salient for the ever-increasing number of older adults today, health literacy is important for all individuals.

The textbook includes chapters that focus on an introduction to the field of health literacy, health literacy strategies across disciplines, and models for use with special, diverse populations. The contributors have shared research, approaches, interventions, and recommendations on increasing health literacy in diverse disciplines. Case studies are embedded throughout the textbook, and a supplemental PowerPoint package, including discussion questions for each chapter, is available for qualified instructors (e-mail: textbook@springerpub.com).

REFERENCES

Centers for Disease Control and Prevention (CDC). (2011). *Older adults: Why is health literacy important?* Retrieved from http://www.cdc.gov/healthliteracy/DevelopMaterials/Audiences/OlderAdults/importance.html

Howard, D. H., Gazmararian, J., & Parker, R. M. (2005). The impact of low health literacy on the medical costs of Medicare managed care enrollees. *The American Journal of Medicine, 118,* 371–377.

Kirsch, I. S., Jungeblut, A., Jenkins, L., & Kolstad, A. (1993). *Adult literacy in America: A first look at the results of the National Adult Literacy Survey (NALS).* Washington, DC: National Center for Education Statistics, U.S. Department of Education.

Ratzan, S. C., & Parker, R. M. (2000). Introduction. In C. R. Selden, M. Zorn, S. C. Ratzan, & R. M. Parker (Eds.), *National Library of Medicine current bibliographies in medicine: Health literacy.* Bethesda, MD: National Library of Medicine, National Institutes of Health.

Scott T. L., Gazmararian, J. A., Williams, M. V., & Baker, D. W. (2002). Health literacy and preventive health care use among Medicare enrollees in a managed care organization. *Medical Care, 40*(5), 395–404.

Weiss, B. D. (2007). *Health literacy: A manual for clinicians* (2nd ed.). Chicago, IL: American Medical Association Foundation.

CHAPTER 1

Health Literacy 101

KAREN KOPERA-FRYE

Health literacy is the degree to which individuals have the capacity to obtain, process, and understand basic health information and services needed to make appropriate health decisions (Ratzan & Parker, 2000). The roots of health literacy can be traced back to the national literacy movement in India under Mohandas Gandhi to assist groups working in foreign countries like Africa to promote health education and promote women's education. The term "health literacy" was first used in 1974 and referred to health education "meeting minimal standards for all school grade levels" (Ratzan, 2001). For the next 30 years various definitions emerged, but all held in common the idea that health literacy involves the need for people to understand information that helps maintain optimal health.

With the increased focus on health literacy programs and research in the 1990s, health literacy evolved into two different approaches. One focused on clinical care and the other on public health (Pleasant & Kuruvilla, 2008). The clinical or biomedical approach often involved the nature of patient–provider interaction with much of the focus on health literacy efforts in the United States and Europe (Pleasant & Kuruvilla, 2008; Sorensen et al., 2013). This approach to health literacy that dominated in the United States in the 1980s to 1990s often depicted individuals, especially older adults, as lacking or suffering from low health literacy, with the underlying assumption that recipients are passive in receiving health information. This approach has produced, and continues to produce, primarily correlated studies (Pleasant & Kuruvilla, 2008). Further, this approach falls short when placed in the broader, more salient ecological, and cultural framework of health.

In contrast, the public health approach to health literacy is more prominent in newly developing nations, where various organizations offer charitable work to provide educational opportunities and improve

1

health for groups in these countries. Although the United States produces most of the research on health literacy (Kondilis, Kiriaze, Athanasoulia, & Falagas, 2008), Europe has strong international programs and research endeavors as well (Brand & Sorensen, 2010). Health literacy experts in developing countries have created successful programs implemented at community levels, EuroHealthNet (Christmann, 2005).

Many factors determine the health literacy levels of educational materials or individuals. Reading level, numeracy level, current health status, language and cultural barriers, cultural relevancy, format of materials, sentence structure, illustration use, and other factors may affect how easily health information is understood and followed. Individual and system factors such as communication levels of both health care provider and patient, lay person's and professional's knowledge of health care topics, demands of the health care and public health systems, and demanding of health care context all affect health literacy levels (Institute of Medicine, 2009, 2013, 2014).

Health literacy affects an individual's ability to communicate effectively one's personal information such as health history with health care providers, effectively participate in patient self-care and chronic disease management programs, understand numerical and/or mathematical concepts involved in probability of risk and medication dosages, and navigate health care information systems. In today's health care systems, patients are responsible for understanding detailed health information, implementing complex medical self-care instructions, and navigating an increasingly complex health care system (e.g., Medicare Part D prescription guidelines). These demands are frustrating and challenging, in many cases even for individuals with high levels of health literacy; for those patients with lower levels, the demands can quickly become overwhelming (Cornett, 2009; U.S. Department of Health and Human Services & Office of Disease Prevention and Health Promotion, 2010).

Health literacy includes various skills that are critical for maintaining health. For example, calculating cholesterol and blood sugar levels for diabetics, measuring and understanding medications, and being able to comprehend nutrition labels, all require math skills. Choosing health plans or comparing prescription drug benefits in plans involves math when calculating premiums, copays, and deductibles. In addition to numerical literacy, health literacy requires basic knowledge of health. Individuals with limited health literacy often lack basic information about body functions and the nature and causes of diseases—information that is critical to understanding health and the impact of lifestyle behaviors such as exercise, smoking, and so on.

Health literacy, according to the Institute of Medicine (2004), is defined as the ability to obtain, understand, and act on health care information and instructions. This definition includes determining when and where to seek health care, understanding and completing health forms and consents (e.g., Health Insurance Portability and Accountability Act [HIPAA], interpreting complex written, and verbal instructions about medication or treatment procedures), and being able to remember and implement these instructions after returning home (aftercare). Many individuals lack basic health literacy to be able to perform these behaviors.

The prevalence of limited health literacy among U.S. adults is estimated to be between 26% and 36% (Kutner, Greenburg, Jin, & Paulsen, 2006; Paasche-Orlow, Parker, Gazmararian, Nielsen-Bohlman, & Rudd, 2005; Sand-Jecklin & Coyle, 2014). The Agency for Healthcare Research and Quality estimates that over 75 million U.S. adults who speak English have limitations in health literacy (Agency for Healthcare Research and Quality, 2011). Lower health literacy is greatest among older adults, individuals with lower educational levels, rural residents (Hoover et al., n.d.; Young, Weinert, & Spring, 2012; Zoellner et al., 2011), ethnically diverse populations, and those living in poverty (Bergsma, 2010; Ginde, Weiner, Pallin, & Camargo, 2008).

In fact, the connection between lower health literacy and the outcome of increasing health disparities among subgroups is a newly emerging area of interest. According to the 2007 Health States Award (Morgan Quinto Press, 2007), the Lower Mississippi Delta region encompassing Arkansas, Louisiana, and Mississippi has the highest rate of health disparities, particularly among African Americans with chronic diseases such as diabetes (Casey et al., 2004; U.S. Census Bureau, 2007). Residents are at the two lowest levels of reading literacy for this region as follows: 64% of Mississippi residents, 61% of Louisiana residents, and 56% of Arkansas residents, as compared to the national illiteracy rate of 46% (Johnson & Strange, 2005). In parishes that border the Mississippi Delta, the percentage of residents functioning at the two lowest levels of proficiency increases to 82%, 78%, and 78%, respectively, for Mississippi, Louisiana, and Arkansas (U.S. Department of Education, Institute of Education Sciences, & National Center for Education Statistics, 2009). Therefore, the link between low health literacy and negative health outcomes is marked in this region.

Another study of 2,600 patients conducted by two U.S. hospitals (Williams et al., 1995) found that between 26% and 60% of the patients could not understand medication directions, a standard informed consent, or basic health care information materials. Limited health literacy has been linked to a host of poorer health outcomes, including increased risk of hospitalization and mortality among older adults (Baker et al., 2002, 2007). A number of other studies have shown that caregivers with low levels of health literacy have difficulties comprehending written materials, may not understand the importance of therapeutic regimes with chronic medical conditions, and may not understand proper use of an inhaler with asthma (Apter et al., 2006; DeWalt, Dilling, Rosenthal, & Pignone, 2007; Williams et al., 1995). Poorer health outcomes and overall health, higher mortality, lower use of preventative health screening services, and increased use of emergency department services have also been linked to lower levels of health literacy (Agency for Healthcare Research and Quality, 2011; Berkman et al., 2014; DeWalt, Berkman, Sheridan, Lohr, & Pignone, 2004; Peterson et al., 2011; Wolf, Gazmararian, & Baker, 2005).

A current approach to examining health literacy and effects of low health literacy views health literacy as an outcome of health promotion (Nutbeam, 2000). This model suggests a hierarchical framework which involves levels of outcome. For example, mortality, morbidity, and disability may represent end-stage health and social outcomes, whereas intermediate outcomes represent the determinants of these health and social outcomes, for example, physical activity or proper nutrition. In this schema, health promotion outcomes involve those personal, social, and structural factors that can be modified to change the intermediate health outcomes; often the goal of healthy lifestyle interventions. Within the framework, health literacy involves the cognitive, social, and personal skills necessary to understand, gain access to, and use the information effectively to support and maintain healthy behaviors. For example, by understanding the importance of physical activity and making the choice to engage in activity, health literacy is increased via health education, thereby influencing the end-stage outcomes. This framework realizes the role of health education and communication in the context of health promotions, while recognizing health literacy also as an outcome of health education. Therefore, health literacy is both influenced by, and an agent of influence on, health promotion education.

According to the Institute of Medicine (2004), low health literacy negatively affects the treatment outcome and safety of care implementation. Patients present in the health care setting with very different levels of health experiences, knowledge or understanding levels, and diverse health literacy skills (Sand-Jecklin, Daniels, & Lucke-Wold, 2016). Having low health literacy can be very frustrating for individuals and dangerous. Research is suggesting that individuals with low health literacy are at higher risk for frequent emergency department visits and readmissions (Cloonan, Wood, & Riley, 2013), lower use of preventative services, and poorer prognoses in chronic illness outcomes (Agency for Healthcare Research and Quality, 2011; Berkman et al., 2011; Peterson et al., 2011). Higher hospital readmission rates have been associated with lower health literacy, especially in the current climate of the Affordable Care Act and reduced hospital payments for over-target readmission rates (Cloonan et al., 2013). Research has indicated that factors contributing to the high rate of hospital readmissions include lower health literacy and ineffective provider communication with patients about aftercare, medications, self-care, and warning signs of worsening health (Markley et al., 2013). Mitchell, Sadikova, Jack, and Paasche-Orlow (2012) found that patients with lower health literacy were 1.7 times more likely to return to the emergency department and also be readmitted compared to those with adequate health literacy as measured by the Rapid Estimate of Adult Literacy in Medicine (REALM).

According to the Centers for Disease Control Health Literacy for Public Health Professionals training (CDC, 2014), it is important that we, as public health professionals, address barriers that can prevent audiences from understanding and acting on vital health and safety messages. The most common barriers include:

- *Use of technical or medical terminology.* Words such as "pandemic," "immunize," "transmit," "influenza," and "prevalence" are examples of words that are often misinterpreted.
- *Reliance on print communication.* Relying on one form disregards the preferences and learning styles of different audiences.
- *Focusing on information rather than actions.* Too often, we focus on what we want the audience to know and not on what they should do.
- *Limited awareness of cultural differences.* They further note that language differences and word meanings can lead to misinterpretation and poor understanding. Improving health literacy skills requires a comprehensive set of strategies that includes those listed as follows. Using these strategies will improve the usability of the health information, making your messages more understandable. They advise: (a) use plain language; (b) use culturally and linguistically appropriate messages; (c) design messages that are participatory and user-centered; (d) evaluate the effectiveness of communications; (e) engage regularly with the communities that are targeted by the communication; and (f) consider the

current literacy level of the intended audience, and design messages based on that level.

The following typical scenarios demonstrate the detrimental health consequences when the health care professional does not explain the nature of the problem and/or diagnoses clearly:

Escorted by his teenage granddaughter, an elderly old (sic) Navajo grandfather was taken to the internal medicine clinic for an infection in his right leg. The granddaughter was fluent in English but had very limited Navajo speaking skills. Speaking in English, the doctor informed the man that the infection in his leg would get worse if he did not take this medication as prescribed. The granddaughter could not translate the scientific concept of infection into Navajo language. The doctor asked one of the nurses for help, and although she tried as much as she could, she also was unsuccessful. The old man, becoming frustrated, just agreed the he understood everything that he had been told. He told the nurse he wanted to have a traditional ceremony performed for him within a couple of days, and for her to tell the doctor. The nurse translated this to the doctor, who restated the importance of taking the medicines. The grandfather insisted he understood, but in fact, because he felt that he did not understand the physician's explanation, he decided to go to a traditional medicine man instead. The medicine man helped him the best he could, but the grandfather's leg had to be amputated, which the doctor ascribed to noncompliance. (Institute of Medicine, 2004, p. 108).

Another case illustrates confusion when the health care professional is not clear:

Mr. G. is a 64-year old man with chronic hypertension, diabetes, a high cholesterol level, and gout. He saw his primary care doctor because his left leg was swollen and painful. His doctor diagnosed an early cellulitis and prescribed an antibiotic to be taken for 10 days. After 4 days, Mr. G. went to the emergency department, unable to walk because of the intense pain and swelling of his entire left leg. His blood sugar and blood pressure were both very high, and he was admitted to the hospital to treat the infection and control his blood pressure. During his emergency department treatment and admission, he was examined by and spoke to four different doctors.

The fifth doctor to take a history and examine Mr. G. discovered that he had taken none of his seven chronic medications, nor the newly prescribed antibiotic given to him when his infection first appeared. Mr. G. explained "You see, I already take 19 pills a day, and when I got another one I got confused about my timing, and I was just so scared I might mess up. My daughter usually helps me with my medicines, but she's been sick and I didn't want to worry her" (Institute of Medicine, 2004, p. 167).

Consider the following case for training physicians from the U.S. Department of Health and Human Services publication entitled, *A Physician's Practical Guide to Culturally Competent Care* (2015):

Despite more than 25 years as a family practice physician, Dr. Brown sometimes feels unsure and isolated in his work in Blueville. It strikes him as ironic, as Dr. Brown had expected to feel more confident and connected in a small-town practice, especially since he grew up in Blueville. When he was young, Dr. Brown's schoolmates and friends were the sons and daughters of European-American farmers and ranchers, like he was. Migrant workers would move through during harvest time, but people measured diversity in the number of crops they planted, not in the range of ethnicity, race, gender, age, religion, or sexual orientation of their neighbors. There was a lot of talk about political correctness on the East Coast, but here politics wasn't the issue. The issue, for him, is how to care for patients when he couldn't understand them, or vice versa. Since he arrived 3 months ago, Dr. Brown has felt stressed about the fact that either people didn't understand him, or they didn't listen to him. How does a conscientious doctor provide good care under circumstances like that? What obligations does he have to his patients? It wasn't just about language either. Some people's approach to, and beliefs about, health and health care simply confounded him. Oh, and the customs! If he had one more Hispanic or Vietnamese woman tell him that her family would eat only traditional food. . .

Dr. Rivera and Dr. Brown have talked a bit about the diversity of the patients in their practice. Even though Dr. Rivera speaks Spanish, she also shares Dr. Brown's concerns about communication. The town, over the past 10 to 15 years, has worked to attract immigrants to ensure that the population could sustain itself, since many long-time residents left farming and moved closer to higher paying jobs in the cities. Many of their patients are Vietnamese or Ethiopian, who brought their own languages and cultures to Blueville. In addition, Dr. Rivera, although Hispanic found that she sometimes misconnected with her Mexican patients. They shared the same language but still held different cultural beliefs.

This is an important tool to help health care professionals learn the issues surrounding cultural/language barriers in the health care setting.

Adults having low health literacy have been found to seek health information less frequently, ask fewer questions of their health care providers, and read pharmacy patient pamphlets about medications less (Katz, Jacobson, Veledar, & Kripalani, 2007; Miller et al., 2010). Studies have indicated that health care providers often think they can identify patients having difficulties with understanding; however, many times patient health literacy skills are overestimated (Jukkala, Deupree, & Graham, 2009; Ohl et al., 2010). Health literacy screening can help the health care professional ascertain what level of understanding is present in the patient. However, this notion is not without its critics, as most argue that health care providers use clear, plain language communication with all patients, without assessing health literacy levels (Paasche-Orlow & Wolf, 2008). While screening may not be feasible, there still is a need to ensure patients are not having particular difficulty with written versus oral instructions. The argument follows that if providers are aware of the aptitude for learning in the patient, they can then explain the information at the level the patient can understand.

In 1999, the American Medical Association convened an ad hoc committee to look at the issue of health literacy. Four areas needing research were recommended: (a) health literacy screening; (b) improving communication with low-literacy patients; (c) cost and outcomes of low literacy; and (d) determining how low literacy affects health (cited in McCray, 2005). It is important to realize that low literacy is not an inherent individual-level problem, but one of society in not making health information and services meet the needs of the public. However, measurement endeavors have focused on screening the individuals' level of literacy.

Several different tools exist to measure the level of health literacy in an individual. These include: (a) The National Assessments of Adult Literacy (NAAL); (b) Health Activities Literacy Scale; (c) REALM, also available in Spanish and a teen version; and (d) Test of Functional Health Literacy in Adults (TOFHLA); (e) Newest Vital Sign; (f) Short Assessment of Health Literacy for Spanish-Speaking Adults (SAHLSA); (g) Stieglitz Informal Reading Assessment of Cancer Text; (h) Medical Achievement Reading

Test; (i) Functional Health Literacy Measure; and (j) Health Literacy Screener. Yet, despite this list, these are better thought of as screening tools, not formal measures of health literacy. Additionally, there are tools that assess reading level, but none of these tools measure health literacy in the context of both the health care system and the patient public (Pleasant, 2009). What is needed in the field is a comprehensive, user friendly, freely accessible, valid measure of health literacy. This would allow health care professionals to understand where their patients are in order to effectively communicate vital health information.

Communication and miscommunication between patient and health care providers have been the focus of numerous studies. Several have examined the ability of patients to understand the terminology used by doctors and nurses (Chapman, Abraham, Jenkins, & Fallowfield, 2003; Cutilli, 2007, Lerner, Jehle, Janicke, & Moscati, 2000; Scott & Wiener, 1984; Spees, 1991). It was found that patients may state that they understand what was being said; when tested for understanding, however, in most cases the facts are incorrect or incomplete. Successful communication on health involves can ask any questions they have for clarification more than understanding terminology, but a conversational style that makes patients feel they are equal in the power relationship between doctors and patients. Doctors are encouraged to assess patients' literacy skills, avoid medical jargon, and inquire about patients' concerns and expectations. Pfizer put out a helpful pamphlet entitled, "Help your patients succeed: Tips for improving communication with your patients" (Pfizer Clear Health Communication Initiative, 2007a, 2007b) that suggests utilizing the Ask Me 3 intervention, using the teach back method, and tips for clear communication. The Ask Me 3 tool involves three questions patients should ask their health care providers: (a) What is my main problem? (b) What do I need to do? and (c) Why is it important for me to do this? Auerbach (2000) suggests patients be collaborators in health care decision making. His results indicate that patients want to be involved to the extent that involvement will increase their chances of a positive outcome, that patients process and retain information better if it relates to their concerns, and that patients generally respond positively to enhanced information provision. Barry (1999) and Berry, Seiders, and Wilder (2003) suggest that patient-centered care is critical and involves a systematic change focusing on patients at the center of the health care system, involving access to information and assistance when it is needed, with appropriate communication technologies.

Given the increased use of Internet for health care information (Nielsen-Bohlman & Institute of Medicine, 2004), Eng (2001) notes the "e-health landscape" promises to "usher in a wealth of innovative solutions for seemingly intractable problems in health and health care." Revere and Dunbar (2001) review a variety of computer-based interventions to enhance communication that include a variety of delivery devices, for example, computer, wireless, and types such as generic, personalized, tailored, and targeted. A mass-produced flier can be personalized by adding a patient's name, whereas targeted interventions are customized for a particular sociodemographic group. Tailored interventions refer to individual-specific information, such as a patient's particular medical history. Kreuter, Lukwago, Bucholtz, Clark, and Sanders-Thompson (2002) discuss "cultural tailoring" in which an intervention takes into account not only sociodemographic characteristics (e.g., one's cultural group values, behaviors, and health beliefs), but also the degree of identification with that cultural group. Gustafson and colleagues (1999) developed comprehensive health enhancement support system (CHESS), a home-based computerized system that provides patients with tailored health information, advice, decision support, and immediate access to health care professionals and other patients. The outcomes were positive, in that patients reported more confidence in their doctors, higher quality of life, and more comfort with their care. However, the literacy demands of these Internet and targeted and tailored information interventions have not been examined.

So, what is recommended in this field to advance knowledge? Training our health care professionals on how to utilize methods to improve client health literacy, for example, a teach back method is a start. Kopera-Frye, Griffin, and Roy (2012) examined knowledge levels of health literacy among 101 intraprofessional health care providers. Professionals, for example, nurses, were from three age groups: (a) young adults aged 22 to 39 years; (b) middle adults aged 40 to 54 years; and (c) older adults aged 55 to 87 years. We examined whether there might be potential age differences in knowledge of health literacy as newer professionals may be more aware, or receive more training on employing strategies in order to increase health literacy among their older clients. Results indicated that there was not a statistically significant difference between age groups; however, the younger and the older adults scored higher on the health literacy quiz compared to middle-aged professionals. So the hope is that we will strive for a health literate society and implement ways to improve health literacy for all.

According to the National Action Plan to Improve Health Literacy, goals of the National Quality Strategy involve: (a) developing and disseminating health and safety information that is accurate, accessible, and actionable; (b) promoting changes in the health care system that improve health information, communication, informed decision making, and access to health services; (c) incorporating accurate, standards-based, and developmentally appropriate health and science information; (d) supporting and expanding local efforts to provide adult education, English-language instruction, and culturally and linguistically appropriate health information; (e) building partnerships, developing guidelines, and changing policies; (f) increasing basic research and development, implementation, and evaluation of practices and interventions to improve health literacy; and (g) increasing the dissemination and use of evidence-based health literacy practices and interventions (The National Academies of Sciences, Engineering, and Medicine, 2015).

Along these same lines, Brach and colleagues (2012) described a health literate organization to be one which makes it easier for people to navigate, understand, and use information and services to take care of their health. Rothman (2015) noted the 10 attributes of a health literate organization: leadership that (a) makes health literacy integral to its mission, structure, and operations; (b) integrates health literacy into planning, evaluation measures, patient safety, and quality improvement; (c) prepares the workforce to be health-literate and monitors progress; (d) includes populations served in the design, implementation, and evaluation of health information and services; (e) meets the needs of populations with a range of health literacy skills; (f) uses health literacy strategies in interpersonal communication and confirms understanding; (g) provides easy access to health information and services; (h) designs and distributes print, audio-visual, and social media content that is easy to understand and follow; (i) addresses health literacy in higher-risk situations, for example, medication directions; and (j) communicates clearly what health plans cover and what individuals have to pay. The ultimate goal is to adapt these principles to all of our community agencies and organizations to create a health-literate society.

REFERENCES

Agency for Healthcare Research and Quality. (2011). *Low health literacy linked to higher risk of death and more emergency room visits and hospitalizations.* Rockville, MD: Press Release.

American Medical Association. (1999). Health literacy: Report of Council of Scientific Affairs. Ad Hoc Committee on Health Literacy for the Council on Scientific Affairs. *Journal of the American Medical Association, 281*(6), 552–557.

Apter, A. J., Chen, J., Small, D., Bennett, I. M., Albert, C., Fein, D. G., . . . Van Horne, S. (2006). Asthma numeracy skills and health literacy. *Journal of Asthma, 43,* 705–710.

Auerbach, S. M. (2000). Should patients have control over their own health care? Empirical evidence and research issues. *Annals of Behavioral Medicine, 22*(3), 246–259.

Baker, D. W., Gazmararian, J. A., Williams, M. V., Scott, T., Parker, R. M., Green, D., & Peel, J. (2002). Functional health literacy and risk of hospital admission among Medicare managed care enrollees. *American Journal of Public Health, 92,* 1278–1283.

Baker, D. W., Wolf, M. S., Feinglass, J., Thompson, J. A., Gazmararian, J. A., & Huang, J. (2007). Health literacy and mortality among elderly persons. *Archives of Internal Medicine, 167,* 1503–1509.

Barry, M. J. (1999). Involving patients in medical decision: How can physicians do better? *Journal of the American Medical Association, 282*(24), 2356–2357.

Bergsma, L. J. (2010). *An analysis of National Rural Health Literacy and Sources of Information.* Paper presented at the annual Health Literacy Research Conference, Bethesda, MD.

Berkman, N. D., Sheridan, S. L., Donahue, K. E., Halpern, D. J., Viera, A., Crotty, K., ... Viswanathan, M. (2011). *Health literacy interventions and outcomes: An updated systematic review: Executive summary, evidence report/technology assessment: Number 199.* Rockville, MD: Agency for Healthcare Research and Quality.

Berry, L. L., Seiders, K., & Wilder, S. S. (2003). Innovations in access to care: A patient-centered approach. *Annals of Internal Medicine, 139*(7), 568–574.

Brach, C., Keller, D., Hernandez, L. M., Baur, C., Parker, R., Dreyer, B., ... Schillenger, D. (2012). *Ten attributes of health literate health care organizations.* Washington, DC: Institute of Medicine.

Casey, P., Horton, J., Bogle, M., Fomby, B., Frosythe, W., Goolsby, S., ... Simpson, P. (2004). Self-reported health of residents of the Mississippi Delta. *Journal of Health Care for the Poor and Underserved, 15,* 645–662.

Centers for Disease Control. (2014). Health literacy training for public health professionals. Retrieved from http://www.cdc.gov/healthliteracy/training/page1613.html

Chapman, K., Abraham, C., Jenkins, V., & Fallowfield, L. (2003). Lay understanding of terms used in cancer consultations. *Psycho-Oncology, 12*(6), 557–566.

Christmann, S. (2005). Health Literacy and Internet: Recommendations to promote health literacy by means of the internet. Retrieved from http://eurohealthnet.eu/sites/eurohealthnet.eu/files/publications/pu_8.pdf

Cloonan, P., Wood, J., & Riley, J. B. (2013). Reducing 30-day readmissions. *Journal of Nursing Administration, 43,* 382–386.

Cornett, S. (2009). Assessing and addressing health literacy. *Online Journal of Issues in Nursing, 14*(12). Retrieved from http://www.nursingworld.org/MainMenuCategories/ANAMarketplace/ANAPeriodicals/OJIN/TableofContents/Vol142009/No3Sept09/Assessing-Health-Literacy-.html

Cutilli, C. C. (2007). Health literacy in geriatric patients: An integrative review of the literature. *Orthopaedic Nursing, 26*(1), 43–48.

DeWalt, D. A., Berkman, N. D., Sheridan, S., Lohr, K. N., & Pignone, M. P. (2004). Literacy and health outcomes: A systematic review of the literature. *Journal of General Internal Medicine, 19,* 1228–1239.

DeWalt, D. A., Dilling, M. H., Rosenthal, M. S., & Pignone, M. P. (2007). Low parental literacy associated with worse asthma care measures in children. *Ambulatory Pediatrics, 7*, 25–31.

Eng, T. R. (2001). *The eHealth landscape: A terrain map of emerging information and communication technologies in health and healthcare.* Princeton, NJ: The Robert Wood Johnson Foundation.

Ginde, A. A., Weiner, S. G., Pallin, D. J., & Camargo, C. A. (2008). Multicenter study of limited health literacy in emergency department patients. *Academic Emergency Medicine, 15*, 577–580.

Gustafson, D. H., Hawkins, R., Boberg, E., Pingree, S., Serlin, R. E., Graziano, F., & Chan, C. L. (1999). Impact of a patient-centered, computer-based health information/support system. *American Journal of Preventive Medicine, 16*(1), 1–9.

Hoover, E. L., Pierce, C. S., Spencer, G. A., Britten, M. X., Neff-Smith, M., James, G. D., & Gueldner, S. H. (n.d.). Relationship among functional health literacy, asthma knowledge and the ability to care for asthmatic children in rural dwelling patients. *Journal of Rural Nursing and Health Care, 12*(2), 30–40.

Institute of Medicine. (2004). *Health literacy: A prescription to end confusion.* Washington, DC: National Academies Press.

Institute of Medicine. (2009). *Measures of health literacy: Workshop summary.* Washington, DC: National Academies Press.

Institute of Medicine. (2013). *Health literacy: Improving health, health systems, and health policy around the world: Workshop summary.* Washington, DC: National Academies Press.

Institute of Medicine. (2014). *Implications of health literacy for public health: Workshop summary.* Washington, DC: National Academies Press.

Johnson, J., & Strange, M. (2005). *Why rural matters 2005: The facts about rural education in the 50 states. Rural School and Community Trust.* Retrieved from http://www.ruraledu.org/articles.php?id=2092

Jukkala, A., Deupree, J., & Graham, S. (2009). Knowledge of limited health literacy at an academic health center. *Journal of Continuing Education in Nursing, 40*, 298–302.

Katz, M. G., Jacobson, T. A., Veledar, E., & Kripalani, S. (2007). Patient literacy and questions-asking behavior during the medical encounter: A mixed-method analysis. *Journal of General Internal Medicine, 22*, 782–786.

Kondilis, B. K., Kiriaze, I. J., Athanosoulia, A. P., & Falagas, M. E. (2008). Mapping health literacy research in the European Union: A bibliometric analysis. *PLOS ONE, 3*(6), e2519.

Kopera-Frye, K., Griffin, K. Y., & Roy, D. (2012, August). *Health literacy knowledge among young-, middle-aged, and older adult Louisiana professionals.* Presented at the annual meeting of the American Psychological Association, Orlando, FL.

Kreuter, M. W., Lukwago, S. N., Bucholtz, R. D., Clark, E. M., & Sanders-Thompson, V. (2002). Achieving cultural appropriateness in health promotion programs: Targeted and tailored approaches. *Health Education Behavior, 30*(2), 133–146.

Kutner, M., Greenburg, E., Jin, Y., & Paulsen, C. (2006). *The health literacy of America's adults: Results from the 2003 National Assessment of Adult Literacy.* Washington, DC: U.S. Department of Education: National Center for Education Statistics.

Lerner, E. B., Jehle, D. V., Janicke, D. M., & Moschati, R. M. (2000). Medical communication: Do our patients understand? *American Journal of Emergency Medicine, 18*(7), 764–766.

Markley, J., Andow, V., Sabherwal, K., Wang, Z., Fennell, E., & Dusek, R. (2013). A project to reengineer discharges reduces 30-day readmission rates. *American Journal of Nursing, 113*(7), 55–63.

McCray, A. T. (2005). Promoting health literacy. *Journal of the American Medical Informatics Association, 12*(2), 152–163.

Miller, M. J., Allison, J. J., Schmitt, M. R., Ray, M. N., Funkhouser, E. M., Cobaugh, D. J., ... LaCivita, C. (2010). Using single-item health literacy screening questions to identify patients who read written nonsteroidal anti-inflammatory medicine information provided at pharmacies. *Journal of Health Communication, 15*, 413–427.

Mitchell, S. E., Sadikova, E., Jack, B. W., & Paasche-Orlow, M. K. (2012). Health literacy and 30-day postdischarge hospital utilization. *Journal of Health Communication, 17*, 325–338.

Morgan Quinto Press. (2007). *Results of the health State Awards: State and city ranking publications.* Lawrence, KS: Author.

National Academies of Sciences, Engineering, and Medicine. (2015). *Health literacy: Past, present, and future: Workshop summary.* Washington, DC: National Academies Press. (2000).

Nielsen-Bohlman, L., & Institute of Medicine (U.S.). (2004). Health literacy: A prescription to end confusion. Washington, D.C: National Academies Press.

Nutbeam, D. (2000). Health literacy as a public health goal: A challenge for contemporary health education and communication strategies into the 21st century. *Health Promotion International, 15*(3), 259–267.

Ohl, M., Harris, A., Nurudtinova, D., Car, X., Drohobyczer, D., & Overton, E. T. (2010). Do brief screening questions or provider perception accurately identify persons with low health literacy in the HIV primary care setting? *AIDS Patient Care and STDs, 10*, 623–629.

Paasche-Orlow, M. K., Parker, R. M., Gaznararian, J. A., Nielsen-Bohlman, L. T., & Rudd, R. R. (2005). The prevalence of limited health literacy. *Journal of General Internal Medicine, 20*(2), 175–184.

Paasche-Orlow, M. K., & Wolf, M. S. (2008). Evidence does not support clinical screening of literacy. *Journal of General Internal Medicine, 23*(1), 100–102.

Peterson, P. N., Shetterly, S. M., Clarke, C. L., Bekelman, D. B., Chan, P. S., Allen, L. A., ... Masoudi, F. A. (2011). Health literacy and outcomes among patients with heart failure. *Journal of the American Medical Association, 305*, 1695–1701.

Pfizer Clear Health Communication Initiative. (2007a). Help your patients succeed: Tips for improving communication with your patients. Retrieved from https:// www.pfizer.com/files/health/help-your-patients.pdf

Pfizer Clear Health Communication Initiative. (2007b). Ask Me 3. Retrieved from http://www.scriptyourfuture.org/hcp/download/worksheet/Ask%20Me%20 3%20-%20Tool%20for%20Patient%20Engagement%20.pdf

Pleasant, A. (2009). Health literacy measurement: A brief review and proposal. In *Measures of health literacy: Workshop summary*. Washington, DC: Institute of Medicine.

Pleasant, A., & Kuruvilla, S. (2008). A tale of two health literacies: Public health and clinical approaches to health literacy. *Health Promotion International, 23*(2), 152–159.

Ratzan, S. C. (2001). Health literacy: Communication for the public good. *Health Promotion International, 16*(2), 207–214.

Ratzan, S. C., & Parker, R. M. (2000). Introduction. In C. R. Selden, M. Zorn, S. C. Ratzan, & R. M. Parker (Eds.), *National Library of Medicine current bibliographies in medicine: Health literacy*, NLM Pub. No. CBM 20000-1. Bethesda, MD: National Institutes of Health.

Revere, D., & Dunbar, P. J. (2001). Review of computer-generated outpatient health behavior interventions: Clinical encounters "in Abstentia." *Journal of the American Medical Informatics Association, 8*, 62–79.

Rothman, R. (2015). Creating health-literate health care delivery. In *Health literacy: Past, present, and future: Workshop summary*. Washington, DC: National Academies Press.

Sand-Jecklin, K., & Coyle, S. (2014). Efficiently assessing patient health literacy: The BHLS instrument. *Clinical Nursing Research, 23*(6), 581–600.

Sand-Jecklin, K., Daniels, C. S., & Lucke-Wold, N. (2016). Incorporating health literacy screening into patients' health assessment. *Clinical Nursing Research.* doi:10.1177/1054773815619592

Scott, N., & Weiner, M. F. (1984). "Patientspeak": An exercise in communication. *Journal of Medical Education, 59*(11), 890–893.

Sørensen, K., Van den Broucke, S., Pelikan, J. M., Fullam, J., Doyle, G., Slonska, Z., . . . Brand, H. (2013). Measuring health literacy in populations: Illuminating the design and development process of the European Health Literacy Survey Questionnaire (HLS-EU-Q). *BMC Public Health, 13*, 948.

Spees, C. M. (1991). Knowledge of medical terminology among clients and families. *Image: Journal of Nursing Scholarship, 23*(4), 225–229.

U.S. Census Bureau. (2007). Trends in major risk factors for cardiovascular disease among adults in the Mississippi Delta Region, Mississippi Behavioral Risk Factor Surveillance System, 2001–2010. *Preventing Chronic Disease, 12*(E21), 1–8.

U.S. Department of Education, Institute of Education Sciences, & National Center for Education Statistics. (2009). National assessment of adult literacy: State and counties. Retrieved from http://nces.ed.gov/naal/estimates/StateEstimates.aspx

U.S. Department of Health and Human Services. (2015). A physician's practical guide to culturally competent care. Retrieved from https://cccm.thinkculturalhealth.hhs.gov/default.asp

U.S. Department of Health and Human Services & Office of Disease Prevention and Health Promotion. (2010). *National action plan to improve health literacy*. Washington, DC: Author.

Williams, M., Parker, R. M., Balar, D. W., Parikh, N. S., Pitkin, K., Coates, W. C., & Nurss, J. R. (1995). Inadequate functional health literacy among patients at two public hospitals. *Journal of the American Medical Association, 274*, 1677–1682.

Wolf, M. S., Gazmararian, J. A., & Baker, D. W. (2005). Health literacy and functional health status among older adults. *Archives of Internal Medicine, 165*, 1943–1944.

Young, D., Weinert, C., & Spring, A. (2012). Home on the range-health literacy, rural elderly, well-being. *Journal of Extension, 50*(3), 1–11.

Zoellner, J., You, W., Connell, C., Smith-Ray, R. L., Allen, K., Tucker, K. L., … Estabrooks, P. A. (2011). Health literacy is associated with healthy eating index scores and sugar-sweetened beverage intake: Findings from the rural lower Mississippi Delta. *Journal of the American Dietetic Association, 111*(7), 1012–1020.

CHAPTER 2

Interpreting and Understanding Lab Results

DENNY G. RYMAN

In February of 2014, the U.S. Department of Health and Human Services mandated a rule that allows patient access to all medical records, including medical laboratory test results (HHS, 2014). The rule was intended to provide patients additional information that would allow for more self-directed informed health care decisions and lifestyle modification. As with any medical information, too much information without some degree of understanding has the potential of being wrongly interpreted and creating unwarranted stress. Therefore, it is important for patients to acquire some basic knowledge regarding information associated with laboratory test results.

Laboratory results can vary from biopsy reports, which would need to be explained by a physician or other medical professional, to printouts that may include specific tests from blood or urine that are reported by numerical values, positives or negatives, or type of bacteria. Usually, normal range values are included with the patient's number or value.

Blood or urine tests provide the physician an enormous amount of information used to diagnose disease and to determine proper functioning of organ systems. They are also used to monitor diabetes and cholesterol levels. Conditions ranging from lupus to leukemia to urinary tract infections are detected by laboratory tests.

Items included on a laboratory report will show the patient's name, an identification number, name and address of the laboratory, test report date, and name of the doctor ordering the test. Other information may include specimen source, date, and time of specimen collection, laboratory accession number, name of test(s) performed, test results, and abnormal test results. Lab reports may draw attention to reports by flagging any value not within normal reference range. Additional information may also flag critical results (life-threatening), which must be reported immediately by the lab to the physician, and units of measurement.

PATIENT PREPARATION

Most laboratory testing is done on blood or urine. Other types of specimens include sputum, cerebral spinal fluid, synovial fluid from joints, or swabs from tissue or areas of the body that are infected by bacteria or other microorganisms. Testing accuracy greatly depends on the proper collection of sample and the strict adherence to fasting requirements. For example, it is best to fast 12 hours before any blood samples are collected, if possible. Nonfasting samples will not be accurate especially when testing for glucose or cholesterol levels. The following sample protocols are important for the patient to have some knowledge of in order to maintain the validity of the test.

HEALTH INFORMATION PORTABILITY AND ACCOUNTABILITY ACT

Patient medical results are covered by the Privacy Rule of the Health Information Portability and Accountability Act (HIPPA) of 1996. The Privacy Rule requires that health care providers and others with medical record access (insurance providers and consulting physicians) protect the privacy of health information, sets limits on the use and release of health records, and empowers patients to control certain uses and sharing of their health-related information (HHS, 2014). Many states also have laws to protect patient privacy and limit the release of genetic and other health information.

VENIPUNCTURE

This is the procedure of drawing blood from a patient. Veins in the elbow are frequently used while veins in the hands can be used when necessary. The following protocol is followed when blood is drawn, and the patient should understand the following:

1. Make sure the phlebotomists or nurse knows your name and the tests that are being ordered.
2. Before the venipuncture, the patient's name should be affixed to the blood collection tube(s).

3. When a vein is found, an antiseptic swab is used to disinfect the puncture area.
4. A tourniquet is tied above the elbow allowing for the selected vein to become more exposed.
5. When the needle is withdrawn from a vein, hold the arm up while applying pressure to the site; this will greatly reduce bruising potential.

URINE COLLECTION

The physician may order a urine sample to determine kidney function and signs of a urinary tract infection. The specimen should always be collected in a clean, dry container, and should always be fresh. For routine testing, a freshly voided, midstream (freely flowing) urine sample should be collected. A first morning sample is preferred as it is the most concentrated. Since contamination of a self-collected urine sample will alter results, especially from bacteria found on the hand, the following will greatly reduce the potential of contamination:

1. Wash hands with soap and water
2. Do not touch the inside of the container provided
3. It is best to clean the genital area with a towelette
4. Begin urination for several seconds then fill the container midstream
5. Insure the container is labeled with name and date

BLOOD TESTS

The most commonly performed hematology test is the complete blood count (CBC) that examines cellular elements in the blood, including red blood cells (RBCs), white blood cells (WBCs), and platelets. The CBC also determines Hgb (hemoglobin) and Hct (hematocrit).

WBC or leukocyte count has a normal range between 4,300 and 10,800 cubic meter per minute (cmm). Usually these numbers are reported as 4.3 to 10.8 cmm. A high WBC value (>10.8) often indicates a bacterial infection. A low WBC value (<4.3) may indicate a viral infection. Abnormal values can also indicate allergic reactions and various types of leukemia. There are five types of WBCs seen on a differential count (blood smear viewed under the microscope by a licensed medical laboratory scientist). One hundred cells are counted to determine the differential count of a CBC, which include neutrophils (40%–60% normal), lymphocytes (20%–40% normal), monocytes (2%–8% normal), eosinophils (1%–4% normal), and basophils (0.5%–1% normal). RBC or erythrocyte count has a normal range between 4.2 and 5.9 million cmm. A low RBC count usually indicates some form of anemia. The size, shape, and content of RBCs are determined in the differential count and a number of diseases can be detected, ranging from sickle cell anemia, vitamin deficiency, to parasitic disease. Hematocrit has a normal range of 45% to 52% for men, and 37% to 48% for women. This test is used to diagnose anemia when the normal values are below the reference range (Stiene-Martin & Lotspeich-Steininger, 1998).

Hemoglobin has a normal range of 13 to 18 g/dL for men, and 12 to 16 g/dL for women. RBCs contain hemoglobin, which gives blood its red color. Hemoglobin transports oxygen from the lungs to the entire body, and returns carbon dioxide to the lungs, which is exhaled. Low levels indicate anemia or some form of chronic bleeding. Hemoglobin values temporarily drop during menstruation, which is considered normal.

Mean corpuscular volume (MCV) has a normal range of 80 to 100 fL. The MCV measures the average volume of RBCs, or the average amount of space each RBC fills. Abnormal values could indicate various forms of anemia and are sometimes used to diagnose chronic fatigue syndrome.

Mean corpuscular hemoglobin (MCH) has a normal range of 27 to 32 pg. The test is used to measure the average amount of hemoglobin in the typical RBCs. Values over 32 could signal anemia, while values under 27 may indicate a vitamin or other nutritional deficiency.

Mean corpuscular hemoglobin concentration (MCHC) has a normal range between 28% and 36%. The MCHC measures the average concentration of hemoglobin in a specific amount of RBCs. An MCHC below 28% indicates anemia, whereas an MCHC above 36% may be used to diagnose a nutritional deficiency of vitamin D or other vitamins and minerals.

Red cell distribution width (RDW) has a normal range between 11% and 15%. This test is used to determine the general shape and size of RBCs. Abnormal values, either high or low, can indicate liver disease, anemia, nutritional deficiencies, and a variety of other health conditions. Platelets have a normal range between 150,000 and 400,000 mL. Platelets play a major role in blood clotting. Too many or too few platelets can alter the clotting process in numerous ways. Platelet counts are routinely used to monitor coagulation therapy medications. Mean platelet volume (MPV) has a normal range of 7.5 to 11.5 fL. This test determines the average size of platelets. Values greater than 11.5 indicate large platelets that could lead to heart attack or stroke. Values lower than 7.5 indicate smaller platelets, which can lead to bleeding disorders.

Another hematology test that may be performed during a routine physical examination is the prothrombin time (PT) and the partial pro-thrombin time (PPT). These tests measure a body's coagulation factors, or how well blood clots. The tests are also used to monitor coagulation therapy medications, such as heparin, warfarin, and coumarin.

The PT has a reference range between 10 and 14 seconds, which means that under laboratory analysis, the blood will clot within the reference time period. The PT is used to monitor warfarin and coumarin therapy. Any prolonged PT beyond the reference range is diagnostic for various coagulation disorders or the need to adjust medications. The PTT has a reference range between 20 and 45 seconds. The test is used to monitor heparin and increased values may indicate coagulation disorders, or autoimmune diseases.

An erythrocyte sedimentation rate (ESR) is usually performed when the physician suspects some type of generalized infection or inflammation. The ESR has a normal range between 0 and 20 mm/hr. Values higher than 30 mm/hr often indicate an inflammation such as arthritis, tuberculosis, hepatitis, or tissue damage. A consistent low value around 0 mm/hr may indicate some form of chronic anemia.

METABOLIC PANEL CHEMISTRY

The chemistry panel or metabolic panel is a routine series of tests used to monitor or diagnose a variety of diseases. This panel is more specific to liver and kidney function but is also used to monitor glucose levels of diabetics. Individual tests that comprise metabolic panels often vary according to ordering preferences of physicians. Alanine aminotransferase (ALT), normals are 8 to 37 IU/L. ALT is an enzyme produced by the liver. Any value greater than 37 may indicate some form of liver damage. Liver damage can result from viral infections such as hepatitis, chrosis stemming from alcoholism, or medications that often damage the liver long term, such as over the counter pain medicines and certain antibiotics (Bishop, Fody & Schoeff, 2013).

For albumin, normal values are 3.9 to 5.0 g/dL. Albumin is a protein made by the liver and is used to diagnose liver or kidney problems when values are evaluated.

For alkaline phophatase (ALP), normal is 44 to 147 IU/L. ALP is an enzyme produced by the liver and bone. Levels greater than 147 signal liver or bone-related diseases. Automobile accident victims can have high ALP values due to bone fractures. The test is also used to determine the healing process of fractures. High ALPs also indicate alcoholic liver damage.

Bilirubin has a normal range of 0.1 to 1.9 mg/dL. Bilirubin is released in the blood stream when RBCs break down or die. This provides information about liver, kidney, and gall bladder function. Generally, the higher the bilirubin, the greater the organ damage. Bilirubin values less than 0.1 indicate anemia.

Blood urea nitrogen (BUN) has a normal range of 10 to 20 mg/dL. This test measures kidney and liver function; BUN values greater than 20 are of particular concern for kidney damage. Slightly elevated levels can be caused by medications and a high-protein diet.

Creatinine has different normal levels according to sex. Women have a range of 0.5 to 1.1 mg/dL; men have a range of 0.6 to 1.2 mg/dL. Creatinine is a waste product that is processed by the kidneys. An elevated creatinine would indicate a kidney function issue. Creatinine and BUN levels are usually used together to better analyze kidney damage.

Glucose (fasting blood sugar) has a normal range of 70 to 99 mg/dL. Elderly patients have normal values slightly higher. High levels of glucose indicate diabetes, while levels around 50 or lower indicate hypoglycemia. Blood sugar levels can be affected by diet (especially sugar soft drinks), stress levels, and medications. It is important to fast at least 6 hours before testing.

Calcium has a normal range of 9.0 to 10.5 mg/dL. Elderly patients have normal lower levels. Calcium above 10.5 can indicate kidney function abnormalities, increased active thyroid glands, lymphoma (a type of leukemia), vitamin D deficiency, and pancreatic disease.

Chloride has a normal range of 98 to 106 mEq/L. High chloride levels indicate dehydration, multiple myeloma, kidney, and adrenal gland disorders. Diets high in salt will also increase chloride levels.

Sodium's normal range is 135 to 145 mEq/L. Sodium is a mineral that regulates water levels and functions in nerve impulses and muscle contractions. High levels can cause cardiac arrhythmia, liver, and kidney disease.

Potassium has a normal range of 3.7 to 5.2 mEq/L. This mineral functions to relay nerve impulses, maintains muscle function, and regulates heartbeats. Low potassium values can result from diet or medications containing diuretics (expels water from the body). A potassium value below 3.0 is considered a critical value that could be life-threatening.

Phosphorus has a normal range of 2.4 to 4.1 mg/dL. Phosphorus is related to calcium and functions in bone health. Values above 4.1 can be due to malnutrition, diuretics, excessive vitamin D, long-term antacid use, alcoholism, and problems with the kidneys or parathyroid glands.

Amylase has a reference range between 95 and 290 IU/L for blood (serum) and 35 to 400 IU/L for urine. A high amylase value is very diagnostic for acute pancreatitis. Amylase values of greater than 1,000 IU/L are not uncommon for pancreatitis. Amylase can also be increased in cases of mumps, peptic ulcers, intestinal obstruction, ruptured ectopic pregnancy, and appendicitis. Lipase has a reference range between 0 and 1.0 U/L and is used to confirm acute pancreatitis when high levels are detected.

LIPID PANELS: CHOLESTEROL AND TRIGLYCERIDES

Lipid panels are a group of tests that measure cholesterol, including high-density lipoprotein (HDL; good) cholesterol and low-density lipoprotein (LDL; bad) cholesterol. The panels also measure triglycerides. High cholesterol and triglyceride levels are risk factors for heart disease and stroke. If the values are too high, diet and exercise may lower the levels, if not, medication is prescribed (Spring, 2001). The normal value for cholesterol is below 200 mg/dL. Borderline high values are 200 to 240 mg/dL. High values are considered to be above 240 mg/dL.

Cholesterol is further tested for fractions called HDL, which is considered the good cholesterol in that risk factors for heart disease and stroke are minimal. HDL cholesterol actually protects against heart disease. LDL is considered the bad cholesterol with higher values directly associated with heart attack and stroke. Any HDL value above 60 mg/dL is not considered a risk factor. An HDL value between 50 and 60 mg/dL is still good, but an HDL value below 40 mg/dL for men and 50 mg/dL for women is considered to be poor as it is associated as a risk factor. Healthy LDL values are below 100 mg/dL. LDL borderline high values range from 130 to 159 mg/dL. High values of LDL are greater than 160 mg/dL. Triglycerides (fats in the blood) have a healthy range between 40 and 160 mg/dL. Values above 160 mg/dL may contribute to heart disease and other health issues.

THYROID TESTING

Thyroid tests are often ordered when patients report symptoms of fatigue, nervousness, or hyperactivity. Unexplained weight gain or loss may also cause the physician to order thyroid tests. A thyroid panel includes testing for five substances including thyroid-stimulating hormone (TSH), total thyroxine (Total T4), free thyroxine (Free T2), total triiodothyronine (Total T3), and free triiodothyronine (Free T3). Normal values for TSH are 0.3 to 3, Total T4 are 4.5 to 12.5, Free T4 are between 0.7 and 2.0, Total T3 range between 80 and 220, and Free T4 range between 2.3 and 4.2. These tests are reported as numbers without measurement values, such as dL/mL, or mEq/L. Any low thyroid test value may indicate some form of hypothyroidism, and high values may indicate hyperthyroidism (Turgeson, 2007).

CARDIAC FUNCTION TESTS

Creatine kinase (CK) is found in all tissue but is in highest concentration in skeletal muscle, heart muscle, and brain tissue. CK values are elevated in skeletal and cardiac muscle, and are very diagnostic for acute myocardial infarction (AMI), commonly known as a heart attack. The normal reference range for CK in males is 46 to 171 U/L and 34 to 145 U/L in females.

When CK levels are greater than 200 U/L, three subset or isoenzyme tests of CK are ordered that include CK-MM (specific for heart damage), CK-MB (specific for skeletal muscle damage), and CK-BB (specific for brain damage). With a heart attack, CK-MM levels will peak in 12 to 24 hours and return to normal within 48 to 72 hours.

Lactate dehydrogenase(LD) enzymes are always ordered with the CK. LD reference range is 125 to 220 U/L. With heart attack, LD values will rise within 12 to 24 hours, peak at 48 to 72 hours, then remain elevated for up to 10 days before returning to normal.

URINALYSIS AND BODY FLUIDS

The most frequently ordered test is the routine urinalysis, which gives the physician a variety of information about the function of the kidneys. Urine is an important testing sample as it contains bodies' waste products. A complete urinalysis is composed of multiple tests, including physical, microscopic, and chemical analysis. Urine testing is routinely used for diabetic monitoring, drug screening (including prescription medications), urinary tract infections, and the initial diagnosis of many diseases which are flagged by abnormal results. As previously mentioned, the proper collection of a urine sample is vastly important in the accuracy of results.

Urine testing involves the use of a test strip (dipstick), which contains reagents that react when certain substances in the urine are present, and a microscopic analysis is performed to view sediment containing bacteria, blood cells, and crystals. A brief summary of test results includes (Leach & Ryman, 2004):

Color: Urine color varies according to diet and medications ingested, but a typical color is a clear yellow. Other colors may indicate blood (red) or green to purple (medications). A cloudy urine may indicate RBCs or WBCs (infection), bacteria, and other formed elements, some of which are normal such as amorphous phosphate crystals. A normal urine has little to no odor, but a bacterial infection will produce a strong odor. Excessive exercise or a high-protein diet (Atkins diet) will produce a sweet or fruity odor. Various other odors are usually attributed to dietary intake and do not indicate disease.

Specific Gravity: This test determines the kidneys' ability to reabsorb essential chemicals and water. The test also determines dehydration and antidiuretic hormone abnormalities. A normal specific gravity ranges from 1.001 to 1.035. Values above 1.035 may indicate liver disease, congestive heart failure, and dehydration due to vomiting or diarrhea. A high value may also be temporary with strenuous exercise.

pH: An important role of kidney function is the regulation of the acid/base balance of the body. The normal pH range is from 4.5 to 8.0. A low pH (acidic) may indicate a high-protein diet or uncontrolled diabetes. A high pH (alkaline) may indicate a urinary tract infection or merely an increased consumption of vegetables.

Protein: A normal urine protein is below 10 mg/dL. A high protein content is often diagnostic for renal disease; however, contamination from prostate, seminal, or vaginal secretions can falsely increase the value. Other causes of protein greater than 10 mg/dL can result from kidney infections or autoimmune disorders such as lupus. Sometimes, an elevated protein value will be temporary resulting from exercise, fever, dehydration, or pregnancy (especially late term).

Glucose: This is used mostly to monitor diabetics or diagnose initial problems with glucose metabolism. A high value can also be due to pregnancy, central nervous system damage, or pregnancy.

Ketones: These are the by-product of fat breakdown. Normal urine contains no ketones but will begin to show up in the urine as a result when fat is not broken down completely or when fat reserves are needed for energy. The presence of ketones indicates a high-protein diet, excessive exercise, dehydration, rapid weight loss, and can be diagnostic for diabetes and other chemical imbalances (sodium or potassium).

Blood: A reagent strip will detect blood or hemoglobin in the urine by a color change of the strip. Blood in the urine can indicate kidney stones, kidney infection, some type of internal trauma, toxins, and pregnancy. In rare cases, strenuous exercise will cause the presence of blood in the urine.

Bilirubin: This substance is from the normal breakdown of hemoglobin when red cells die. Too much bilirubin in the blood may result from hepatitis, cirrhosis, gall stones, or early liver disease.

Urobilinogen: This is a bile pigment from hemoglobin breakdown, which is indicated by a color change on the reagent strip. An increase of urobilinogen in the urine can indicate bacterial infections, and early liver disease.

Nitrate: This is a quick test for a urinary tract infection but can also indicate cystitis and pyelonenephritis. The test is often used for the evaluation of UTI antibiotic therapy. A positive test is indicated by a color change on the urine reagent strip.

Leukocytes: A positive leukocyte test indicates WBCs in the urine. When combined with a positive nitrate test, is diagnostic for a urinary tract infection.

A microscopic analysis of the urine sample is performed when one or more of the reagent strip tests are positive. The urine is placed under the microscope to determine what formed element is present. These formed elements can include:

RBCs: The number of cells may be reported as ranging from few to numerous. The presence and amount of blood is directly related to the bleeding that is occurring.

WBCs: A microscopic analysis is performed to confirm a positive reagent strip test. This usually indicates a urinary tract or kidney infection.

Epithelial Cells: These are cells that line the urogenital tract areas. Their presence can be normal (squamous) to more indicative of disease as when transitional or renal tubular epithelial cells are seen.

Casts: These formed elements are unique to the kidney and different casts represent various clinical conditions.

Crystals: These are another formed element found in the kidney that are formed by the precipitation of urine salts. The formation of urine crystals is enhanced when urine flow is inhibited through the kidneys.

A specialized urine test is mandated by law to be performed on newborns. The phenylketonuria (PKU) test detects a gene failure to produce an essential enzyme used by the body to break down certain foods. This rare syndrome affects 1 in 10,000 births and if undetected will result in severe mental retardation. If the PKU is positive, the child will be placed on a restricted diet for several years until the body begins to produce the enzyme as the child grows (Shimeld, 1999).

Several additional tests are not routinely ordered in the physician's or clinic office but the patient should understand basic information derived from body fluids and stool samples.

Seminal fluid (sperm) is evaluated with cases of infertility or post-vasectomy. Collection of the sample is important as the container must be sterile, the sample must be obtained after a 3-day period of no sex, the sample cannot be collected in a condom (contain spermicidal agents) and must be taken to the lab within 1 hour of testing at room temperature. Any value outside the normal for sperm analysis could be a sign of infertility. Seven characteristics are reported when sperm are evaluated, including volume (2–5 mL), viscosity (liquefied vs. clumpy), appearance (clear), pH (7.2–7.8), sperm count (20–160 million/mL, less than 10 million/mL is considered sterile), motility (a grade of 3 or 4 is used to describe proper motility or movement), and shape (abnormal forms are double-tailed, giant headed, or other abnormal shapes).

Fecal analysis is used to detect gastrointestinal bleeding, colon cancer (bloody stool), liver disorders, and bacterial, viral, or parasitic infections. Color and consistency are important in fecal analysis as black (tarry) stools indicate GI bleeding, watery stool indicated diarrhea, and ribbon-like stools indicate possible obstruction. The occult blood test is a simple quick test where a small stool sample is placed on paper containing a chemical that reacts with blood; if blood is present, a blue color will form.

Other body fluids are ordered only when a specific disease or condition is suspected. Amniotic fluid, a protective fluid that surrounds a fetus, is used for genetic testing of the fetus. Pleural or pericardial fluid, which surrounds the heart, may be drawn to determine infection. Cerebrospinal fluid (CSF) is analyzed to diagnose possible meningitis. All body fluids, including urine, are normally sterile.

IMMUNOLOGY AND SEROLOGY

Any test that uses antibodies (what the body produces) and antigens (what the body produces against foreign substances like viruses) reactions in testing for various diseases generally falls under the immunology or serology category. Most immunology/serological testing is ordered only for specific diseases but may be ordered routinely when patient symptoms are generalized or vague.

Hepatitis testing uses the ELISA process (automated serological analysis performed by lab instrumentation) to detect a rise in titer, or how many antibodies the body is producing in response to the hepatitis virus. There are several variants of hepatitis but the most common types are Hepatitis A (HAV), Hepatitis B (HBV), and Hepatitis C (HCV). Early detection is important in fighting the disease as hepatitis (Hepatitis C) is usually fatal if untreated (Shimeld, 1999).

Hepatitis A is transmitted by the fecal-oral route, with food or water contamination usually the cause. Mortality rates are less than 1%, but liver damage can result. Recovery from Hepatitis A infection occurs within 2 to 4 weeks. Vaccines are available for HAV.

Hepatitis B is transmitted when contaminated blood comes in contact with another person through needle sticks, tattooing, ear piercing, or contaminated blood transfusions. Sexual transmission also occurs when one partner has the virus. The infection can last up to 6 months before recovery with moderate to severe liver damage resulting. Liver cancer has been linked to Hepatitis B.

Hepatitis C is transmitted like Hepatitis B, but sexual transmission is less common. Hepatitis C is more chronic in nature and is fatal if untreated. A vaccine has recently been approved by the Food and Drug Administration and new medicines have been developed to treat the disease.

HIV causes AIDs. Testing is by detecting antibodies to HIV and HIV antigens. Numerous home testing kits are available using a sample of saliva; the test indicates only a negative or positive reaction. More specific laboratory tests will confirm a negative or positive quick test result. Laboratory result reports vary by state and may include a simple negative or positive to more involved results giving the percentages and ratios of T-Cells and other leukocytes (WBCs). Physician consultation is necessary in understanding individual results (Mahon & Manuselis, 2000).

Other routine serological tests using quick test methodology (results are immediate) are used to diagnose mono (mononucleosis) caused by the Epstein–Barr virus, Lyme disease caused by Borrelia Burgdorferi bacteria, and the common quick Strep test used to detect a Strep B throat infection. Less frequent serological testing is done for suspected cases of Rocky Mountain Spotted Fever, mycoplasma pneumonia, Legionnaires' disease, and Chlamydia pneumonia.

MISCELLAN SPECIFIC TESTS (CANCER TUMOR MARKERS)

There are literally thousands of laboratory tests that can be ordered by a physician. Ordering nonroutine tests requires the physician to have a particular reason for ordering due to third-party insurance provider payment. The following miscellaneous tests, although still not part of routine blood work, are frequently ordered to rule in or rule out a particular disease or condition. They become more frequent when monitoring treatment protocols.

Tumor markers are substances that are produced by the body in response to cancer, or produced by the cancer itself. Some of these markers are specific to one particular cancer, while others are seen in several different types of cancer. Tumor markers are generally used to evaluate the patient's response to treatment or to monitor for recurrence (when cancer returns after treatment). There are noncancerous conditions that can elevate markers, so results must be interpreted by the physician. Tumor markers are often used in conjunction with other tests to help diagnose a patient who has symptoms suspicious for cancer. Some markers can help the physician determine prognosis and treatment (Skirton, Christine & Williams, 2004).

Tumor markers are not elevated in all cases of the cancers with which they are normally associated, and they are not helpful in all patients. For example, carcinoembryonic antigen (CEA) is used to detect colon cancer recurrence, yet it is produced in only 70% to 80% of colon cancer cases. In addition, only 25% of cases that are limited to the colon (early stages) have elevated CEA. Therefore, it cannot always detect colon cancer in its early stages, when cure rates are best. Tumor markers can be very helpful in following response to treatment and recurrence, but they cannot replace physical examination, evaluation of symptoms, and radiologic studies.

Prostate specific antigen (PSA) has a normal range of 0 to 4 ng/mL. A test is diagnostic for prostate cancer when values are elevate, and also is used to monitor treatment. Other conditions that can elevate values are infections of the prostate, or any type of injury or trauma to the prostate.

Cancer antigen 125 (CA 125) has a normal range of 0 to 35 U/mL. A test is used to monitor treatment and recurrence of ovarian, breast, colorectal, uterine, cervical, pancreatic, liver, or lung cancer. Noncancer high values can be caused by pregnancy, menstruation, endometriosis, pelvic inflammatory disease, and liver disease, especially hepatitis.

Cancer antigen 27.29 (CA 27.29) has a reference range of less than 40 U/mL; levels greater than 100 U/mL signify cancer. It is used to detect recurrence or metastasis of breast cancer. Noncancerous high values include liver and kidney disorders, and benign breast problems.

The normal range for carcinoembryonic antigen (CEA) is less than 2.5 ng/mL in nonsmokers, and less than 5.0 ng/mL in smokers. Values over 100 ng/mL signify metastatic cancer. It is used to test for a variety of cancers including colorectal, breast, lung pancreatic, thyroid, cervical, ovarian, liver, head and neck, and melanoma. Noncancerous high values can be caused by cigarette smoking, hepatitis, pancreatitis, peptic ulcers, and hypothyroidism.

Bence-Jones proteins have a normal range of 0.00 mg/dL. A value of 0.03 to 0.05 mg/dL is significant for early detection of cancer. The test is used for initial diagnosis of multiple myeloma or chronic lymphocytic leukemia. Urine is the specimen of choice. There are no known noncancerous rises in values.

Cancer antigen 15.3 (CA 15.3) has a reference range of less than 31 U/mL. It is used to monitor treatment and recurrence of breast cancer. However, it is not sensitive enough during early stages of breast cancer. It is also used to detect lung, ovarian, endometrial, bladder, and gastrointestinal cancers. Noncancerous elevations include liver disease, lupus, sarcoid, and noncancerous breast lesions.

Cancer antigen 19.9 (CA 19.9) has a reference range of less than 37 U/mL, and values greater than 120 U/mL are generally indicative of tumor development. It is used in the detection and monitoring of pancreatic, colorectal, liver, and stomach cancers. Inflammation and thyroid disease can result in elevated values.

The reference range for thyroglobulin (Tg) is 0 to 33 ng/mL. If the entire thyroid is removed, the normal range is 0 to 2 ng/mL. Tg is used to detect thyroid cancer and to monitor treatment and possible recurrence. There are no known noncancerous causes for elevated levels.

The alpha-fetoprotein (AFP) reference range is 0 to 15 IU/mL for both men and women. Values greater than 400 IU/mL indicate cancer. AFP is diagnostic for testicular and ovarian cancer. Higher values can also be caused by pregnancy (AFP clears after birth), liver disease, and inflammatory bowel disease.

Human chorionic gonadotrophin (HCG) has a normal range in men of less than 2.5 U/mL. In nonpregnant women, the range is less than 5.0 U/mL. HCG is used to diagnose testicular cancer and some precancerous growths in women. HCG levels are also used to determine pregnancy, and are used in home testing pregnancy kits. Noncancerous elevated levels are caused by pregnancy, marijuana use, cirrhosis of the liver, duodenal ulcers, and inflammatory bowel disease.

Calcitonin is a tumor marker for some forms of thyroid cancer with a reference range of less than 8.5 pg/mL for men, and less than 5.0 pg/mL for women. Noncancerous elevated values can be caused by kidney disease, and the use of medications given to reduce stomach acid.

GENETIC TESTING FOR HEREDITARY CANCER SYNDROMES

Genetic testing is not normally part of routine blood work and is usually ordered by specialists only when a patient's medical history indicates a potential for cancer development in future years. Genetic testing looks for specific inherited changes (mutations) in a person's chromosomes, genes, or proteins. Genetic mutations can have harmful, beneficial, neutral (no effect), or uncertain effects on health. Genetic testing is done to determine whether family members without obvious illness have inherited the same mutation as a family member who is known to carry a cancer-associated maturation.

There are more than 50 hereditary cancer syndromes for which testing can be done. The majority of these are caused by mutations that are inherited from close family members. Even if a cancer-predisposing mutation is present in a family, it does not necessarily mean that everyone who inherits the mutation will develop cancer. Genetic counseling by experts in the field is available when patients have questions about their results or even if they should be tested at all. The following is an abbreviated list of hereditary genes that are the most common when genetic testing is ordered (Skirton, Christine & Williams, 2004).

> BRCA1 and BRCA2 are genes related to breast cancer in both men and women, and ovarian cancer.
>
> TP53 genes are associated with a number of cancers including: breast, bone, leukemia, brain, and adrenal.
>
> PTEN genes are associated with breast, thyroid, and endometrial cancer.
>
> MSHE, MLH1, MSH6, PMS2, EPCAM are a group of genes that are collectively known as "Lynch syndrome" genes. They are related to colorectal, endometrial, ovarian, renal pelvic, pancreatic, small intestine, liver, brain, and breast cancers.

APC genes are associated with colorectal, nonmalignant colon polyps, brain, stomach, bone, and skin cancers.

RB1 is related to retinoblastoma or eye cancer.

VHL, also known as "Von Hippel–Lindau syndrome," is related to kidney cancer and multiple noncancerous tumors.

Medical test results are normally included in a person's medical records. Therefore, people considering genetic testing should understand that their results may become known to other people or organizations that have legitimate, legal access to their medical records, such as their insurance company or employer.

In 2008, the Genetic Information Nondiscrimination Act (GINA) became federal law for all U.S. residents. GINA prohibits discrimination based on genetic information in determining health insurance eligibility or rates and suitability for employment. However, GINA does not cover members of the military, and it does not apply to life insurance, disability insurance, or long-term care insurance.

SUMMARY

Basic knowledge of laboratory test results, including proper sample collection methods, are important when patients want to better understand their medical or physical conditions. But it is important to note that a diagnosis of a specific condition requires many factors including medical history, radiographic (x-ray, MRI, etc.), and other testing avenues available to medical professionals. Patient knowledge about results and diseases is always important in discussions with physicians. Various websites are available to the public that can provide additional information to the patient about a particular laboratory test used to diagnose a specific disease or condition. In conclusion, the medical professional should be consulted for detailed information about laboratory test results because an elevated test result may be insignificant when combined with the entire report.

REFERENCES

Bishop, M. L., Fody, E. P., & Schoeff, L. E. (2013). *Clinical chemistry, principles, techniques, and correlations* (7th ed.). Philadelphia, PA: Lippincott Williams & Williams.

Leach, D. L., & Ryman, D. G. (2004). *Outline review of medical technology/clinical laboratory science*. Upper Saddle River, NJ: Prentice Hall.

Mahon, M. R., & Manuselis, G. (2000). *Textbook of diagnostic microbiology* (2nd ed.). Philadelphia, PA: Saunders.

Shimeld, L. A. (1999). *Essentials of diagnostic microbiology.* Boston, MA: Delmar.

Skirton, H. B., Christine, P. C., & Williams, J. R. (2004). *Applied genetics in healthcare.* New York, NY: Garland Science.

Spring, K. R. (2001). *Clinical laboratory tests* (2nd ed.). New York, NY: Springhouse.

Stiene-Martin, E. A., Lotspeich-Steininger, C. A., & Koepke, J. A. (1998). *Clinical hematology, principles, procedures, correlations* (2nd ed.). Philadelphia, PA: Lippincott.

Turgeson, M. L. (2007). *Clinical laboratory science: The basics and routine techniques* (5th ed.). St. Louis, MO: Elsevier.

U.S. Department of Health and Human Services (2014). HHS strengthens patients' right to access lab test reports. Retrieved from http://www.federalregister.gov.

CHAPTER 3

Physician Approaches to Increasing Patient Health Literacy

SAMER N. ROY, SHREYA SAHAY SAXENA, AND KRISHNAKANT SHAH

In the United States, the population over age 65 has tripled across the last 30 years (U.S. Census Bureau, 2014). As a result, the standard of medical practice will be greatly influenced by the health care needs of older individuals. Geriatric assessment differs from a typical medical evaluation by including both medical and nonmedical domains (e.g., widowhood). It requires the physician to assess an older patient's physical ability and cognition, extensively review prescription medications, review immunization status, diagnose medical conditions (acute or chronic), develop treatment and follow-up plans, coordinate care management, and evaluate long-term care needs and optimal living placement. Within a busy clinical practice, effectively evaluating geriatric patients can be quite challenging for a physician. This chapter is designed to share ways the physician can explain the diagnosis and treatment regimen to older patients, thereby increasing patient health literacy.

In order to fully appreciate the differences in serving an older versus younger patient, it is necessary for us to understand the physiological processes associated with the aging process. Aging results in senescent or normal changes in cognition such as slower processing of information. Other specific changes that occur with aging include reduced vision, hearing capacity, greater tendency to be distracted, and reduced capacity to process and remember new information. Often, the older population may have a multitude of health problems that are often chronic, progressive, debilitating, and comorbid (e.g., diabetes and hypertension). Physicians need to prepare for an increasing number of older patients by developing a greater understanding of this population and developing enhanced communication with these patients.

Special consideration in working with older patients includes disease manifestation, perceptions of illness, heavy medication usage, and diversity among them. Disease symptoms may be masked in older patients. Confusion, for example, may be the only symptom of an infection, hypoxia, or cerebrovascular accident. Pain is often an unreliable symptom because some older patients seem to lose pain perception and experience pain in a different manner from other patients. The excruciating pain usually associated with pancreatitis, for example, may be perceived by the older patients as a dull ache. Occasionally, myocardial infarction can occur without chest pain. Falls are the sixth leading cause of death for older people and a contributing factor in 40% of admissions to nursing homes. Falls in elderly patients are rarely due to a single cause as a seemingly minor fall may be due to a serious problem such as urinary tract infection, smoldering pneumonia, or transient ischemic attack (TIA). Thus, establishing a diagnosis and effective prevention of disease progression requires a more thorough comprehensive assessment of the patient's medical condition.

Additionally, the elderly have more adverse reactions to medications, in large part due to altered pharmacokinetics and pharmacodynamics. Commonly used drugs such as digoxin have prolonged half-lives, and central nervous system tissues may become more sensitive to certain drugs such as benzodiazepine and narcotics. The tendency for multiple problems to be treated with multiple drugs places the older adults at risk for iatrogenic disorders. A complete medication history is essential, with special attention given to the interaction of drugs and communicating specific information regarding dosage to the individual.

One of the biggest problems physicians face when dealing with older patients is that they are actually more heterogeneous than younger patients. Their wide range of life experiences and cultural backgrounds often influence their perceptions of illness, willingness to adhere to medical regimens, and ability to communicate effectively with health care providers. Strangely, when older patients have the greatest need to communicate with their physicians, life events, and physiologic changes may make it challenging. The primary responsibility for improving health care facilities for older adults lies with health care professionals, in many cases, the primary care physician. Lack of communication between physician and patient has been linked to poor health outcomes such as higher rates of hospitalization and less frequent use of preventive services. An important consideration should always be effective communication of health care information. Approaches that physicians can keep in mind while explaining the diagnosis and treatment regimen to their geriatric patients include aspects of plain language (Kutner, Greenberg, Jin, & Paulsen, 2006).

PLAIN LANGUAGE ... Keep it simple

Avoid long or run-on sentences. Do not use medical or technical terms that are difficult for the patient to understand. Organize similar information into several smaller groups. As a general guide, use no more than four main messages. Speaking in plain language boosts understanding for older adults, even with a possible cognitive impairment.

Focus on Important Details

Because patients may search for meaning in everything you say, avoid being careless by giving extra information. When communicating with them, stay focused on important details. Personalize information only when necessary and minimize distractions. Be sure details such as timing and the order of health-related treatment actions are understood. The critical thing for them to understand is the order and timing of various medications to be taken.

Written Set of Instruction

Providing an information sheet that summarizes the most important points of the visit and explains what the patient needs to do after he or she leaves your office is important. Ask the patient to post the written instructions on the refrigerator or a bulletin board so that the instructions remain fresh in his or her mind. The written cues will reinforce the oral directions given.

Watch the Patient's Facial Expressions

It is also important to recognize that the patient–physician interaction involves a two-way exchange of nonverbal information. Patients' facial expressions are often good indicators of sadness, worry, or anxiety. The physician who responds with appropriate concern to these nonverbal cues will likely have a greater positive impact on the older patient's illness as compared to the physician wanting to strictly convey factual information. At the very least, the attentive physician will have a more satisfied patient.

Repeat Essential Information

All patients will benefit from repetition of important information. The physician should emphasize and keep repeating the health information until the receivers are able to restate the information given. Specifically, ask them to act out the medication regimen while in the office.

Be a Good Listener

A slower pace of speech may be needed when working with older adults. Listening with patience, as well as encouraging them to speak, leads to increased understanding. Calmly and patiently listening to them will convey ease and may encourage them to speak more about their problems. Some elderly patients suffer from depression; maybe as many as 10% of a caseload (Park & Unutzer, 2011). The more they offer to tell you about how they are feeling, the closer you may get to an appropriate diagnosis.

Slow Down Rate of Speech

Physicians who provide information in a slow and deliberate fashion allow the time needed for patients to comprehend the new information. Other techniques physicians can use include pausing frequently and reinforcing silence with appropriate body language. One study found (Traveline, Ruchinskas, & D'Alonzo, 2005) that physicians typically wait only 23 seconds after a patient begins describing his or her chief complaint before interrupting and redirecting the discussion. Such premature redirection can lead to late-arising concerns and missed opportunities to gather important data.

Be Empathetic

Empathy is a basic skill all physicians should practice; not just for elderly patients, but for patients of all age groups. Physicians should not ignore or minimize patient feelings with a redirected line of inquiry relentlessly focusing on "real" symptoms. Patient satisfaction is likely to be enhanced by physicians who acknowledge patients' expressed emotions (Stewart, 1995).

Ask for Written Patient List of Complaints

Recollection of all issues ailing the older patient may prove difficult for some patients. Physicians should advise the patients to keep a list of their complaints to be addressed during the doctor visit.

Use the "Teach Back" Method

Teach back involves the health care provider asking the person receiving the information to restate it. This method fosters understanding, promotes comprehension, and may show areas not clearly understood. Teach back is an example of an evaluation strategy for in-the-moment education to access the recall and comprehension of the patient. Essential considerations of teach back include evaluation of language proficiency and language barriers, literacy levels, sensory impairments, evidence of dementia, delirium, or depression, and use of key terms at critical times (Tamura-Lis, 2013). Teach back also has been shown to be effective in patients with low literacy to help them understand privacy and confidentiality (Kripalani, Bengtzen, Henderson, & Jacobson, 2008).

Be Sensitive to Patient Needs

Not every older adult is the same, and not every older adult will experience significant mental decline. Some elder patients need help in a specific area, such as short-term memory so look for ways to clarify those needs to facilitate understanding. Whereas some medical conditions can result in permanent changes in executive function, be aware of the effects of illness and recovery. Physicians should be competent in explaining to the patient all health care information. For example, for a patient who is suffering from terminal stage cancer, the possibility of hospice care and/or home health nurse care should be clearly discussed. The first step for the physician is to focus on the response, allowing sufficient time for a full display of emotions, and then talking about the patient's feelings.

Use of Medical Devices

If a medical device such as an oxygen tank is important to a patient's health, the physician needs to make sure it is used appropriately. Thoroughly explaining the steps involved and employing pictures or drawings can facilitate understanding. The physician should also be able to assess the patient's capability to use the device, possibly even in situations of stress.

Role of Caregiver

Asking older adult patients to bring their caregivers with them to the appointments is extremely helpful. Although most older patients are able to comprehend the health-related information their physicians want to convey, some may suffer from memory loss or confusion. For these patients, explaining the care plan to both the patient and caregiver becomes critical.

Easy to Read Fliers

Fliers that are developed by the Centers for Disease Control and Prevention are an ideal form of written information for older adults. Physicians can use charts, models, or pictures to help the patient understand his or her condition and treatment (Weiss, 2007). These fliers are available in multiple languages. Fliers prepared in English will not necessarily help individuals who do not have English as their primary language. Fliers in various languages are a better way to ensure understanding among a diverse group of patients.

Give Patients an Opportunity to Ask Questions and Express Themselves

Once treatment has been explained and all necessary information has been provided, patients should have ample opportunity to ask questions. This allows them to express any apprehensions they might have or clear up any misunderstandings.

Older Patients With Sensory Losses

Some degree of hearing loss is not uncommon in the later years. For patients suffering hearing loss, the physician should take a position in front of the patient, speaking clearly and slowly, taking care not to shout.

Shouting only magnifies the problem by distorting the consonants and vowels. In many cases, a written explanation may ultimately be less frustrating for both physician and patient. If this becomes necessary, tailor the process to include the most pertinent questions, because this method can be tedious and exhausting for patients. Conversely, impaired visual perception and light-dark adaptation can adversely affect the process of explaining information as well. Provide the patient with a well-illuminated environment and a light source that does not glare or reflect in the eyes. This illuminated surrounding leads to less distraction for the patient.

The ultimate benefit of applying these communication techniques will be improvement in outcomes for older patients and caregivers (Marshall, 2015). Research indicates that outcomes of health care for older adults are dependent not only on biomedical needs, but also on the caring relationship created through effective communication (Hingle & Robinson, 2009). With effective physician–older patient communication, patients are more likely to share their symptoms and concern, which will enable the physician to make a more accurate diagnosis. Additionally, patients are more likely to follow through with the physician recommendations, less likely skip appointments, and will be more likely to talk to the physician if they want to switch their medication because of the side effects or perceived nonefficacy. Research has indicated that if such communication skills are applied, older patients are more apt to adhere to preventive care for their chronic diseases. Other research reports (Bertakis & Azari, 2011) decreased diagnostic testing cost as a function of better physician–older patient communication.

As opposed to younger patients, interviews with older adult patients in themselves can be therapeutic. The physician–older patient relationship goes beyond medical care, and instead is based on trust and comfort. An important element in this relationship is open and frequent communication between the physician and older patient. One review of clinical randomized controlled trials on patient–physician communications reported that the quality of communication in the history-taking and management-discussing portions of the interactions influenced patient outcomes in 16 of 21 studies. Outcomes influenced by such communication included emotional health, symptom resolution, function, pain control, and physiological measures such as blood pressure level or blood sugar level. The review identified specific elements of effective communication. For example, patient anxiety was reduced in patients whose physicians encouraged questions, and shared in the decision-making process (Stewart, 1995).

Research indicates that patient–doctor communication factors affect patient satisfaction and outcomes such as medication compliance (Laine et al., 1996; Like & Zyzanski, 1987; Robbins et al., 1993). Patient–doctor communication is also enhanced by utilizing a patient-centered approach to interviewing (Smith & Hoppe, 1991), which involves considering the patient's perception of his or her illness as just as valued as the physician's diagnostic goal. Elements of this communication style include: not interrupting patients' opening statements; using facilitating comments—for example, "Is there anything else?" or "uh-huh" to discover the patient's full range of concerns; and actively listening to the patient's story (Beckman, Markakis, Suchman, & Frankel, 1994; Brown, Weston, & Stewart, 1989) by paying attention to his or her emotional state and making empathic statements; soliciting the patient's perception—for example, "What do you think is going on?"—which allows for the physician's understanding of the patient's primary concerns; and establishing agreement on the goals of visits and treatment by involving patients in their own care (Beckman et al., 1994). It was found by Roland, Bartholomew, Courtenay, Morris, and Morrell (1986) that physicians who increased their average office visit length from 6.7 to 7.4 minutes (face-to-face) asked more questions related to health history and psychosocial concerns and had a greater understanding of treatment among their patients.

Today's managed care environments present more challenges to, and opportunities for, effective communication and maintenance of the patient–physician relationship (Council on Ethical and Judicial Affairs, 1995; Emanuel & Dubler, 1995; Gordon, Baker, & Levinson, 1995; Irby, 1995). Trainees need to be taught effective communication skills in this environment that include: (a) enhanced patient–doctor communication for time management, which involves using charting and face-to-face and non-face-to-face visit time efficiently; (b) following an experienced doctor and seeing that he or she touches lab reports results and other clinical reports once by reading and acting on them; (c) helping patients deal with the uncertainty in their medical conditions or concerns, for example, progression of cancer; and (d) viewing physician time as a resource to maximize the patient–doctor relationship.

ROLE OF THE AMERICAN FAMILY PHYSICIAN IN GERIATRIC CARE

The following discusses specific geriatric issues that most likely the physician will face when working with older adults: assistive devices, elder mistreatment, failure to thrive, fall prevention, geriatric assessment, house calls, impaired visual acuity, and nursing home care. New research may affect the interpretation and application of this material; however, physician's clinical judgment is essential for implementation of the following (Greene & Johnson, 1993).

Geriatric Assessment

The geriatric assessment is a multidimensional assessment designed to evaluate an older person's functional ability, physical health, cognition and mental health, and socioenvironmental circumstances (Spaulding & Sebesta, 2008). It includes an extensive review of prescriptions, as most of the medicines are chronic, and over-the-counter drugs, vitamins, and herbal products, as well as a review of immunization status. It is essential for the physician to detect a potential problem such as confusion, falls, immobility, or incontinence. However, older persons often do not present in a typical manner, and atypical responses to illness are common. A patient presenting with confusion may not have a neurologic problem, but rather an infection. Social and psychological factors may also mask classic disease presentations. For example, although 30% of adults older than 85 years have dementia, many physicians miss the diagnosis. In such cases, patients prove to be poor historians, and careful assessment is critical in such cases. While assessing patients, topics such as nutrition, vision, hearing, fecal and urinary incontinence, balance, and fall prevention should be kept in mind.

Functional Ability

The physician should be able to assess an individual's functional capability, which has two key divisions: activities of daily living (ADL) and instrumental activities of daily living (IADL). ADL are self-care activities that a person performs daily, such as eating, dressing, bathing, transferring between bed and chair, toileting, bladder control, and bowel functions. IADL are activities that are needed to live independently such as doing housework, preparing meals, taking medications, managing finances, and using the telephone. For details, refer to the Katz Index of Independence in ADL (Katz, 1983; Katz, Doun, Cash, & Grotz, 1994). Physicians can simply acquire information by observing older patients as they complete tasks in the clinic itself, like unbuttoning and buttoning a shirt while preparing for a physical exam.

Nutritional Assessment

At later ages, the intake of food is compromised. Causes for reduced food intake may include loneliness-related depression, mood disorders leading to loss of appetite, generalized weakness, and dyspepsia. A nutritional assessment is important because inadequate micronutrient intake is common in older persons. Several age-related medical conditions may predispose patients to vitamin and mineral deficiencies. Studies have shown that vitamins A, C, D, and B_{12}, calcium, iron, zinc, and other trace minerals are often deficient in the older population. During the physical examination, particular attention should be given to signs associated with inadequate nutrition and a 24-hour food diary should be obtained (Elsawy & Higgins, 2011).

Physical Activity

According to the American College of Sports Medicine (ACSM, 1998), aerobic and muscle-strengthening activities are critical for healthy aging. Recommendations include moderate intensity aerobic activity and muscle strengthening exercises for 2 hours and 30 minutes in a week. For details, refer to the recommendations for physical activities in older adults by ACSM. The physician's role is to convince older patients to adopt a physically active lifestyle. This has several benefits, foremost being body mass index control. Obesity, in itself, is a major contributory factor to many medical ailments, such as osteoarthritis, diabetes mellitus type 2, falls, debility, and so forth. A study reported that life expectancy was even increased in a person who didn't begin exercise until he was 75 years of age (Elsawy & Higgins, 2010). During the office visit, the physician should stress the importance of physical activity and introduce exercise options and guidelines. Physicians may provide a take-home information packet including handouts on exercise-associated health benefits, resistance, aerobic, and flexibility training, and lifestyle modification (McDermott & Mernitz, 2006).

Detecting Elder Abuse and Neglect

There are several types of elder abuse: financial or material, neglect or abandonment, physical, psychological, emotional, or sexual (World Health Organization [WHO], 2006). The National Center on Elder

Abuse defines elder abuse as "intentional or neglectful acts by a caregiver or 'trusted' individual that lead to, or may lead to, harm of a vulnerable elder." One out of 10 older adults experience some form of abuse or neglect each year and the incidence is expected to increase. The Elder Abuse Suspicion Index (EASI) was validated in a primary care setting and can be used by physicians to screen cognitively intact patients during routine visits (Hoover & Polson, 2014). While assessing for suspected elder abuse, physicians must differentiate disease processes or normal aging from signs of injuries. Underlying conditions that mimic intentional injury or predispose the patient to injury should be noted. Adverse reactions to home remedies and prescription and nonprescription medications can resemble intentional injuries. Physicians should interview the patient alone, if abuse is suspected. Physicians in most states have a legal and professional obligation to accurately diagnose and report any unexplained bruise marks, bruises, or fractures. Family physicians will need to involve local social services and Adult Protective Services (APS) to determine options for the older abused patient.

Balance and Fall Prevention

Falls are the leading cause of injury in the elderly population (Croswell & Shin, 2013). For effective primary care intervention for falls, the physician can use various approaches to identify persons at increased risk. However, no evidence-based instrument exists that can accurately identify older adults at increased risk of falling. The U.S. Preventive Services Task Force (USPSTF, 2012) found convincing evidence that exercise or physical therapy has moderate benefit in preventing falls in older adults (Mathias, Nayak, & Isaacs, 1986). A clinical summary of the USPSTF Recommendations for Prevention of Falls in a community-dwelling elderly population should be followed. These include what primary care clinicians can reasonably consider a small number of factors to identify older persons at increased risk for falls. Age itself is strongly related to risk for falls (Rakel, 2000; Seidel, Ball, Davis, & Benedict, 1999). Several clinical factors including a history of falls, a history of mobility problems, and poor performance on the timed Get-Up-and-Go test (Hill, 1998; Kelly, 1997; Podsiadlo & Richardson, 1991) also identify persons at increased risk for falling. A history of falling is most commonly used to identify increased risk for future falling and has generally been considered concurrently or sequentially with other key risk factors, particularly gait and balance. The test is performed by observing the time it takes a person to rise from an armchair, walk 3 m (10 ft.), turn, walk back, and sit down again (Kelly, 1997). The average healthy adult older than 60 years can perform this task in less than 10 seconds (Greene, Johnson, & Lemcke, 1998). The USPSTF did not report evidence involving frequency of a brief falls risk assessment, but other organizations, including the American Geriatric Society (AGS), recommend that clinicians ask their patients yearly about falls and balance or gait problems. Physicians caring for older adults should inquire at least annually about falls, and should inquire about and examine their difficulties with gait and disbalance while observing for any dysfunction. The older patient can benefit from use of canes or a walker, if used appropriately.

Driving Problems

Physicians should routinely ask about driving status. The automobile is the most important form of transportation for older adults, and the ability to drive is a key element in maintaining independence. However, individual autonomy in driving must be balanced with public safety. A range of medical problems can affect the ability of older adults to drive safely such as cognitive impairment, including dementia (Carr, 2006). Cognitive impairment is defined as a decline in at least one of the following domains: short-term memory, attention, orientation, judgment and problem-solving skills, and visuospatial skills. Referral for performance-based road testing may further clarify the potential risk and assist in making driving recommendations. Physicians should assist families in the difficult process of driving cessation, including providing information about websites and other resources in addition to clarifying appropriate state regulations. The Older Drivers Project sponsored by the American Medical Association (AMA) developed office-based assessments of functional abilities related to driving, a reference table of medical conditions with safety recommendations for several diseases, recommendations for counseling patients on driving cessation, and a discussion of the legal and ethical issues associated with the care of unsafe drivers. These tools are available in the *Physician's Guide to Assessing and Counseling Older Drivers* (AMA, 2010), which was created by the AMA with support from the National Highway Traffic and Safety Administration. This guide addresses many aspects of older adult driving and can be used in the office by physicians.

Failure to Thrive

Unintentional weight loss in older patients can drastically affect their ability to perform day-to-day activities, increase debilities and hospitalizations, and overall mortality. Unintentional weight loss (i.e., more than 5% reduction in body weight in less than 6 months) can be attributed to malignant causes, nonmalignant gastrointestinal problems, or psychiatric disorders. Polypharmacy in adults interferes with taste and causes anorexia; some medications cause dry mouth, dysphagia, and or nausea. Other causes of anorexia in elder patients may be isolation and depression. Physicians should identify the cause for weight loss by running a series of blood tests and imaging, and rectify the problem. This often involves a multidisciplinary team, including dentists, dietitians, speech, occupational, or physical therapists, and social service workers. Starting the patient on appetite stimulants can help (Thomas, 2011).

Polypharmacy

Most elderly patients are on antithrombotics, antihypertensives, antidiabetics, and antidepressants medications at the same time. Common, but serious manifestations of polypharmacy include falls, orthostatic hypotension, delirium, gastrointestinal bleeds, and so forth. While the physician does not always have the option of discontinuing the medications, strategies can be designed to reduce the risk of adverse drug events. Beers et al. (1991), Screening Tool of Older Persons' Prescriptions (STOPP), and Screening Tool to Alert Doctors to Right Treatment (O'Mahony et al., 2010) criteria can help identify problem-causing drugs. Since it takes longer for older adults to metabolize medications, this requires certain drugs to be given in much lower doses than usual. Another risk of polypharmacy in adults is their impaired cognition, which can lead them to over- or underdose certain medicines. Medication reconciliation should be done every visit by the physician, and in case of any discrepancy, pharmacies should be contacted to verify medications and the frequency with which they have been filled.

Home health visiting nurses and family members can monitor the taking of medications to prevent trouble.

Cancer Screening

Physicians should discuss the potential benefits and dangers of screening for cancer with every patient. Cancer is the second leading cause of death in elderly patients in the United States, making cancer screening necessary. Colonoscopy, mammograms and prostate-specific antigen (PSA) level testing can help to detect cancers early in the course, potentially increasing life expectancy.

Screening for Hearing Loss

Pure tone audiometry, in primary care clinical practice, may be used to evaluate any potential hearing deficits when hearing loss is suspected in a patient. As a part of a preventive approach, physicians may consider placing educational materials on hearing loss prevention in their waiting rooms and inquiring if there are problems during the visit (Walker, Cleveland, Darris, & Seales, 2003).

Screening for Vision

Impaired visual acuity is a serious public health problem in the elderly. The USPSTF found evidence that early treatment of refractive error, cataracts, and age-related macular degeneration improves or prevents loss of visual acuity. However, there was inadequate evidence that treatment improves functional outcomes. Therefore, early screening is critical. Assessing vision during the office visit is necessary for early prevention of visual problems.

Nursing Home Care

Nursing home care is a complex, highly regulated, and dynamic process. The combination of chronic health conditions and increased need for assistance with ADL leads to special medical, social, behavioral, and spiritual needs. One and a half million people aged 65 years in the United States have spent some time in a nursing home and 51% of nursing home residents require assistance with all ADL. The most common diseases in nursing home residents include mental disorders or those involving the circulatory or central nervous system. Nursing homes vary greatly in size and scope of services. They may provide short-stay care, posthospitalization rehabilitation for community-dwelling patients, and hospice care. More than 80% of nursing homes use community physicians to provide care, but they also may employ staff physicians or contract with physician groups. Correct timing of elderly assessment and transferring the patient to a nursing home depends on the family and physician. The family should be counseled on the most suitable placement for their loved one.

Pain Management in the Elderly

Pain is a common subjective experience for many older adults, and is often associated with a number of chronic (e.g., osteoarthritis) and acute (e.g., cancer, surgery) conditions. Despite its prevalence, evidence suggests that pain is often poorly assessed and poorly managed, especially among older adults. Cognitive impairment, due to dementia and/or delirium represents a particular challenge to pain management because older adults with these conditions may be unable to verbalize their pain. Simple choices in words, information depth, speech patterns, body position, and facial expression can greatly affect the quality of one-on-one communication between the patient and physician. Avoiding communication pitfalls and sharpening the basic communication skills previously suggested can help strengthen the bond that many patients and physicians believe is lacking.

A report by the Gerontological Society of America (GSA, 2012) and another from the National Institute on Aging (2008) offer recommendations on how physicians and other health professionals can best communicate with older patients. They suggest the following: (a) avoid speech that might be seen as patronizing, (b) recognize the tendency to stereotype older patients; (c) control nonverbal behavior and use direct, concrete, and actionable language; (d) use humor and a direct communication style with caution with patients of non-Western cultures; (e) face the patient while speaking, using pictures and diagrams for clarifying information about the disease; (f) ask open-ended questions and pay attention to sentence formation; (g) ask about the patient's living condition to rule out elderly abuse; (h) avoid making ageist assumptions; (i) engage the patient in decision making; and (j) express understanding and compassion, which are the bases for all conversation skills. The physician should help patients coping with chronic diseases by finding reputable sources of online and community support. Physicians and other health professionals should always have a positive tone while interacting with elderly individuals. Effective doctor–patient communication is a central clinical function in building a therapeutic doctor–patient relationship, which is the heart and the art of medicine. Doctors and other health professionals must work together to ensure that health information and services can be understood and used appropriately by one and all.

REFERENCES

American College of Sports Medicine. (1998). Exercise and physical activity for older adults. *Medical Science Sports Exercise, 30*(6), 992–1008.

American Medical Association. (2010). *Physician's guide to assessing and counseling older drivers.* Retrieved from http://www.ama-assn.org/go/olderdrivers

Beckman, H., Markakis, K., Suchman, A., & Frankel, R. (1994). Getting the most from a 20-minute visit. *American Journal of Gastroenterology, 89,* 662–664.

Beers, M. H., Ouslander, J. G., Rollingher, I., Reuben, D. B., Brooks, J., & Beck, J. C. (1991). Explicit criteria for determining inappropriate medication use in nursing home residents. Archives of Internal Medicine, 151(9), 1825–1832.

Bertakis, K. D., & Azari, R. (2011). Patient-centered care is associated with decreased health care utilization. *Journal of the American Board of Family Medicine, 24*(3), 229–239.

Bohannon, R. W. (2006). Reference values for the timed up and go test: A descriptive meta-analysis. *Journal of Geriatric Physical Therapy, 26*(2), 64–68.

Brown, J. B., Weston, W. W., & Stewart, M. A. (1989). Patient-centered interviewing II: Understanding patients' experiences. *Canadian Family Physician, 35,*153–157.

Carr, D. B. (2006). *Older adult drivers with cognitive impairment.* Retrieved from http://www.aafp.org/afp/2006/0315/p1029

Council on Ethical and Judicial Affairs. (1995). Ethical issues on managed care. *Journal of the American Medical Association, 273,* 330–335.

Croswell, J. M., & Shin, Y. (2013). Prevention of falls in community-dwelling older adults: 48–56. Recommendations statement. *American Family Physician, 86*(12), 1135–1136.

Elsawy, B., & Higgins, K. E. (2010). Physical activity guidelines for older adults. *American Family Physician, 81*(1), 55–59.

Elsawy, B., & Higgins, K. E. (2011). The geriatric assessment. *American Family Physician, 83*(1), 48–56.

Emanuel, E. J., & Dubler, N. N. (1995). Preserving the physician-patient relationship in the era of managed care. *Journal of the American Medical Association, 273,* 323–329.

Gerontological Society of America. (2012). *Communicating with older adults: An evidence-based review of what really works*. Retrieved from http://www.lasell.edu/Documents/talk-of-ages/GSA_Communicating-with-Older-Adults-low-Final.pdf

Gordon, G. H., Baker, L., & Levinson, W. (1995). Physician-patient communication in managed care. *Western Journal of Medicine, 163*, 527–531.

Greene, H. L., & Johnson, W. P. (1993). *Decision making in medicine* (2nd ed.). St. Louis, MO: Mosby.

Greene, H. L., Johnson, W. P., & Lemcke, D. P. (1998). *Decision making in medicine: An algorithmic approach*. St. Louis, MO: Mosby.

Hill, M. G. (1998). The practice of medicine. In A. S. Fauci & D. L. Longo (Eds.), *Harrison's principles of internal medicine*. New York, NY: McGraw-Hill.

Hingle, S. T., & Robinson, S. (2009). Enhancing communications with older patients in the outpatient setting. *Seminar in Medical Practices, 12*, 1–7.

Hoover, R. M., & Polson, M. (2014). Detecting elder abuse and neglect: Assessment and intervention. *American Family Physician, 89*(6), 453–460.

Irby, D. M. (1995). Teaching and learning in ambulatory care settings: A thematic review of the literature. *Academy of Medicine, 70*, 898–931.

Katz, S. (1983). Assessing self-maintenance: Activities of daily living mobility, and instrumental activities of daily living. *Journal of the American Geriatrics Society, 37*, 267–271.

Katz, S., Doun, T. D., Cash, H. L., & Grotz, R. C. (1994). Progress in development of the index of ADL. *Gerontologist, 10*, 20–30.

Kelly, W. N. (1997). Humanistic qualities in medicine. In R. Winters & M. B. Murphy (Eds.), *Textbook of internal medicine* (3rd ed.). Philadelphia, PA: Lippincott-Raven.

Kripalani, S., Bengtzen, R., Henderson, L. E., & Jacobson, T. A. (2008). Clinical research in low-literacy populations: Using teach-back to assess comprehension of informed consent and privacy information. *IRB: Ethics Human Research, 30*(2), 13–19.

Kutner, M., Greenberg, E., Jin, Y., & Paulsen, C. (2006). *The health literacy of America's adults: Results from the 2003 national assessment of adult literacy* (NCES–483). U.S. Department of Education. Washington, DC: National Center for Education Statistics.

Laine, C., Davidoff, F., Lewis, C. E., Nelson, E. C., Nelson, E., Kessler, R. C., & Delbanco, T. L. (1996). Important elements of outpatient care: A comparison of patients' and physicians' options. *Annals of Internal Medicine, 125*(8), 640–645.

Like, R., & Zyzanski, S. J. (1987). Patient satisfaction with the clinical encounter: Social psychological determinants. *Social Science Medicine, 24*, 351–357.

Marshall, L. C. (2015). Nurses as educator within health system. *Mastering patient and family education: A healthcare handbook for success*. Indianapolis, IN: Sigma Theta Tau International.

Mathias, S., Nayak, U. S., & Isaacs, B. (1986). Balance in elderly patients: The "get-up and go" test. *Archives of Physical Medicine and Rehabilitation, 67*, 387–389.

McDermott, A. Y., & Mernitz, H. (2006). Exercise and older patients: Prescribing guidelines. *American Family Physician, 74*(3), 437–444.

National Institute on Aging. (2008). *A clinician's handbook: Talking with your older patient*. Retrieved from www.nia.nih.gov/.../default/files/talking_with_your_older_patient.pdf

O'Mahony, D., Gallagher, P., Ryan, C., Hamilton, H., Barry, P., O'Connor, M., & Kennedy, J. (2010). STOPP AND START criteria: A new approach to detecting potentially inappropriate prescribing in old age. *European Geriatric Medicine, 1,* 45–51.

Park, M., & Unutzer, J. (2011). Geriatric depression primary care. *Psychiatric Clinics of North America, 34*(2), 469–487

Podsiadlo, D., & Richardson, S. (1991). The timed "Up & Go": A test of basic functional mobility for frail elderly persons. *Journal of the American Geriatrics Society, 39,* 142–148.

Rakel, R. E. (2000). Pain Management. In R. R. Kersey & L. Gery (Eds.), *Saunders manual of medical practice.* Philadelphia, PA: W. B. Saunders.

Robbins, J. A., Bertakis, K. D., Helms, L., Azari, R., Callahan, E. J., & Creten, D. A. (1993). The influence of physician practice behaviors in patient satisfaction. *Family Medicine, 25,* 17–20.

Roland, M. O., Bartholomew, J., Courtenay, M. J. F., Morris, R. W., & Morrell, D. C. (1986). The "five minute" consultation: Effect of time constraint on verbal communication. *British Medical Journal, 292,* 874–876.

Seidel, H. M., Ball, J. W., Dains, J. E., & Benedict, G. W. (1999). Comparison of value orientation among cultural groups. In J. Thompson & G. Brower (Eds.), *Mosby's guide to physical examination.* St. Louis, MO: Mosby.

Smith, R. C., & Hoppe, R. B. (1991). The patient's story: Integrating the patient-and physician-centered approaches to interviewing. *Annals of Internal Medicine, 115,* 470–477.

Spalding, M. C., & Sebesta, S. C. (2008). Geriatric screening and preventive care. *American Family Physician, 78*(2), 206–215.

Stewart, M. A. (1995). Effective physician-patient communication and health outcomes: A review. *Canadian Medical Association Journal, 152*(9), 1423–1433.

Tamura-Lis, W. (2013). Teach-back for quality education and patient safety. *Urologic Nursing, 33*(6), 267–271.

Thomas, D. R. (2011). Use of orexigenic medications in geriatric patients. *American Journal of Geriatric Pharmacotherapy, 9*(2), 97–108.

Traveline, J. M., Ruchinskas, R., & D'Alonzo, G. E. (2005). Patient-physician communication: Why and how. *Journal of the American Osteopathic Association, 105,* 13–18.

U.S. Census Bureau. (2014). An aging nation: The older population in the United States. Retrieved from http://census.gov/prod/2014 pubs/ page 25-1140.Pdf

U.S. Preventive Services Task Force. (2012). Prevention of falls in community-dwelling older adults: U.S. preventive services task force recommendation statement. *Annals of Internal Medicine, 157*(3), 197–204.

Walker, J. J., Cleveland, L. M., Darris, J. L., & Seales, J. S. (2013). Audiometry screening and interpretation. *American Family Physician, 87*(1), 41–47.

Weiss, B. D. (2007). *Health literacy and patient safety: Help patients understand: Manual for clinicians.* Chicago, IL: American Medical Association.

World Health Organization. (2006). Elder abuse and alcohol fact sheet. Retrieved from http://www.who.int/violence_injury_prevention/violence/world_report/factsheets/ft_elder.pdf

Adding Value to Physical Therapy With Health Literacy Tools and the Explanatory Model

MARY K. MILIDONIS, JANE G. KEEHAN, AND ALEXANDRA TALBOTT-WELCH

Health care is evolving to meet the needs of an aging population with chronic conditions. The new focus of health care is shifting to the health of populations, the health care experience, and the cost of care (Institute for Healthcare Improvement, n.d.). Individuals with lower health literacy tend to use health care services that are more costly. Lower health literacy is associated with poor outcomes, greater difficulty managing chronic health conditions, and increased mortality (Berkman, Sheridan, Donahue, Halpern, & Crotty, 2011; Koh et al., 2012). Because one-third to one-half of people has difficulty with health literacy, the best course may be to offer accessible health information and health services to everyone (Brega et al., 2015). Recent federal policy initiatives are prioritizing changes in health literacy to improve health care for everyone (Koh et al., 2012). Improvements include spoken communication, written communication, and self-management (Brega et al., 2015).

Health literacy is the ability of someone to understand and engage in his or her own health care. How can health care providers improve health literacy? A synthesis of health literacy research suggests four actionable goals that include improvements in written communication, spoken communication, self-management and empowerment, and supportive systems (Brega et al., 2015).

Effectiveness of rehabilitation that aims to improve functional abilities and health behaviors may be minimized by low health literacy (Ennis, Hawthorne, & Frownfelter, 2012). Low health literacy predicts functional decline in older adults (Smith et al., 2015). Decline in physical function is associated with falling difficulties and cognitive difficulties (Serper et al., 2014). Older adults in physical and occupational therapy may struggle with mobility training, functional tasks, and safety instructions. Using tools to improve health literacy may improve health, safety, and self-management for persons with activity limitations (Brega et al., 2015). Self-management and health enhancement programs are known to improve functional outcomes, exercise tolerance, decrease hospitalizations, and improve quality of life (Dossa & Capitman, 2012). Health care providers using communication tools will hopefully simplify care, minimize confusion, and promote better patient self-management.

UNIVERSAL HEALTH LITERACY INTERVENTION

Low literacy is associated with stigma and poor self-esteem (Mackert, Donovan, Mabry, Guadagno, & Stout, 2014). Low health literacy is easily concealed from health care providers. Concealing stigmatizing low health literacy may lead to poor treatment outcomes (Mackert et al., 2014). Differentiating which patients have low health literacy is difficult for many reasons. Using health literacy tools with every patient is recommended to facilitate treatment adherence, improve outcomes, and minimize costs of care. Universal health literacy intervention precautions are taken to minimize risk that any patient has difficulty understanding instructions (Brega et al., 2015). We have to assume that patients just don't understand our interventions unless proven otherwise. Improving communication includes shared decision making, personalized self-management tools, and building support networks (Brega et al., 2015).

PATIENT PRACTITIONER COLLABORATIVE MODEL

Working collaboratively improves health literacy, patient-centered care, and patient receptivity to change (Jensen, Lorish, & Shepard, 2002). The therapeutic process is more than examination and intervention. It involves the therapist's understanding of the patient's belief system and mediating the patient's belief system with the therapist's own beliefs. Collaborative problem solving and negotiation between the patient and therapist are necessary to find mutually agreeable goals or destination and the path forward. Treatment adherence data suggest that patients are not always dutiful to what they are prescribed. There are many influences on behavior, and knowledge and motivation are only two of many variables that influence treatment adherence. Therapists know that they are more likely to achieve patient adherence when they try to understand the patient's perspective about the condition and its effects. Following a treatment plan requires the patient choosing to follow the plan, knowing when to enact the plan, having the psychomotor skills to perform the plan, and remaining motivated to continue until the problem resolves (Jensen et al., 2002).

Adherence and Health Literacy

Health literacy developed for physicians and pharmacists out of a need to insure adherence to medication interventions. For physical therapists, understanding tools to improve exercise adherence is key to improved patient outcomes. If a patient fails to follow or incorrectly follows a home exercise program (HEP) or postsurgical precautions, he or she will be at risk for injury. Poor adherence could increase the likelihood of falls, post-surgical complications, or the development of chronic disease (Sjosten et al., 2007). Low health literacy can lead to poor communication between physical therapist and patient and limited patient understanding and retention. If a patient leaves the hospital or outpatient clinic with a HEP that he or she does not understand, value, or remember, the likelihood that the patient will adhere to the plan of care may be decreased. Lack of adherence may translate to higher health care costs, increased risk, and poor outcomes (Lascar et al., 2014). Following is a review of exercise adherence facilitators and barriers with a focus on older adult balance exercise programs.

Researchers have examined different aspects of adherence to exercise programs and therefore reported variable adherence rates. For example, some studies compare the frequency of exercise prescribed to the frequency with which the patient performed it, while others compare duration or intensity prescribed to what was performed. Some studies recruit healthy subjects while others recruit subjects with chronic diseases. Some studies include all the patients who enroll in a study, including those who drop out during the trial period, while others report only on patients who complete the entire trial. Some studies of adherence rely on patient report, while others use more objective measures like exercise class attendance. All of these differences in the study of adherence have created a wide range of adherence rates, ranging from 40% to 95% (Rhodes & Fiala, 2009) among the general adult population and from 54% to 78% among older adults (Flegal, Kishiyama, Zajdel,

Haas, & Oken, 2007; Martin & Sinden, 2001). Long-term adherence rates have been observed to drop after the first 6 months of initiating the program (Briggs et al., 2011). Fall prevention HEP adherence rates from 1 to 4 years after initiating the program have been reported from 44% to 58% (Campbell, Robertson, Gardner, Norton, & Buchner, 1999; Forkan et al., 2006).

Exercise adherence research focuses on patient characteristics or beliefs as predictors of, barriers to, or facilitators of adherence. Commonly found predictors of adherence include baseline depression, baseline fatigue, physical health-related quality of life (Flegal et al., 2007), stage of change regarding exercise, age, intention (Courneya et al., 2003), better physical condition, a physically active lifestyle, being a nonsmoker, and higher exercise self-efficacy (Forkan et al., 2006; Martin & Sinden, 2001). In a year-long fall prevention program, lower age, lower self-perceived fall risk, and better physical function at baseline all predicted better adherence. Another study of older adults following a HEP up to 4 years after going through a fall prevention program, found that only barriers and not the motivators studied were predictive of adherence. The most significant predictor in this study was a change in health status. Other predictors included no interest, weather, depression, weakness, fear of falling, shortness of breath, and low outcome expectations (Forkan et al., 2006). In a study of exercise barriers and facilitators for subjects with type 1 diabetes mellitus, they frequently cited a lack of time, lack of access to facilities, lack of motivation, weather conditions, negative feelings about body image, and a lack of understanding about the link between blood sugar and activity (Lascar et al., 2014).

There is a body of research evaluating the link between adherence and interventions. Some intervention strategies found to facilitate adherence among older adults include asking patients about their health beliefs, learning style, and barriers to beginning an exercise program (Ennis et al., 2012). In a systematic review of adherence studies, it was shown that patients were more likely to adhere if they enjoyed the physical activity, received positive feedback from the physical therapist, and collaborated with their physical therapist on overcoming barriers and planning the how, when, and where of the physical activity (Rhodes & Fiala, 2009).

Incorporating self-management strategies appears to increase adherence rates, according to another large systematic review of adherence studies. Some examples of self-management strategies used in conjunction with exercise therapy include setting goals, writing contracts, and educating patients about their disease, managing symptoms, nutrition, emotional coping skills, and relaxation skills. According to the research on interventions to facilitate adherence, physical therapists should consider implementing self-management strategies, assessing learning style, discussing barriers and benefits to exercise, discussing health beliefs, and selecting activities that the patient finds enjoyable.

Closing the gap between the health care provider and the patient is fundamental to improving health literacy. Understanding the perspective, knowledge, and learning style of the patient allows the therapist to assure that the patient understands the health problem and has control over the plan of care. This approach can help to overcome barriers created by low health literacy and facilitate long-term adherence to the HEP. In a survey of physical therapists, only 34.9% screened patients for illiteracy (Billek-Sawhney, Reicherter, Yatta, & Duranko, 2012). Health literacy includes not only literacy, but also listening skills, health knowledge, reading fluency, memory, and the ability to navigate health care environments (Ennis et al., 2012). If the therapist is able to address health literacy by improving patients' understanding of their problems, belief that they are capable of affecting their problems (self-efficacy), and belief that their mutually agreed upon plan is achievable and effective, patients will be more likely to adhere to that plan and to achieve their goals.

Kleinman's Explanatory Model

The success of health care literacy hinges on the comfort level at which clinicians and health care providers can effectively communicate. Communication can be achieved by both written and verbal methods. It is important to remember that each patient/client has his or her own community or network (Plack & Driscoll, 2011), which includes family, friends, significant others, social networks, and more. This network can create both barriers as well as supports. In order to assess a patient/client's readiness to learn and potential adherence to the therapeutic intervention, it is important to clearly communicate. This section will review the Explanatory Model which can facilitate communication with the patient/client.

Dr. Arthur Kleinman is an accomplished American psychiatrist who is well known for his work in medical anthropology and cross-cultural psychiatry at Harvard University. Kleinman is famous for his research which was conducted in China in the late 1970s. He authored the book *Patients and Healers in the Context of Culture* (Kleinman, 1980). Kleinman formulated the term "explanatory model," to describe how both the caregiver and the patient/client may perceive any occurrence of his or her current illness or health. Kleinman's premise was that the health care provider may perceive the patient/client's episode of illness or health much differently than the patient/client. This could be problematic for trying to develop a therapeutic relationship and patient adherence to treatment and intervention. Kleinman suggested that there is a model to facilitate open, clear, and effective communication between the caregiver and the patient/client. He identified that there are two aspects of sickness: disease and illness.

"Disease" refers to dysfunctional biological and/or psychological processes. It also affects individuals and individual perceptions. "Illness," in contrast, refers to the psychosocial experience and takes into account how the dysfunction is affecting the patient/client's social and community networks. Both of these aspects need to be addressed when communicating with the patient/client. The explanatory model allows for this type of communication.

Kleinman's explanatory model explores five major health areas. They are as follows:

- Etiology
- Time and mode of onset of symptoms
- Pathophysiology
- Course of sickness (acute, chronic, etc., degree of severity)
- Treatment

Kleinman suggests the use of eight questions (Kleinman, Eisenberg, & Good, 1978) to clarify and identify the information outlined earlier in the five major health areas. These questions are as follows:

1. What do you call the problem?
2. What do you think has caused the problem?
3. Why do you think it started when it did?
4. What do you think the illness does? How does it work?
5. How severe do you think your illness is? Do you believe it will have a short or long course?
6. What kind of treatment do you think you need? What results do you expect from treatment?

7. What major problems has this illness caused for you?
8. What do you fear most about this illness?

These questions can allow us a "glimpse" into the patient/client's understanding and ability. It allows the health care provider to actively listen and suspend judgment. It is a step toward understanding the patient/client's biases, and cultural and health beliefs. This is the first step in the process of developing a "therapeutic alliance" (Fuentes et al., 2014). It is important to have a mutual relationship in which the goals in our plan of care are patient-centered goals and not practitioner-centered goals. These questions, when used effectively, can also glean meaningful information in regard to the patient/client's health literacy. The questions can help us to determine if there are any misunderstandings or misconceptions about his or her disease or illness. It is important to understand and proceed in a therapeutic relationship in which there is a partnership in which the patient/client takes an active role in health and wellness.

The explanatory model can help practitioners move from using solely the biomedical model to transitioning to using the biopsychosocial model. The biomedical model had been the dominant force in Western medicine since the early 20th century. This model emphasizes a focus on physical processes such as pathology, chemistry, and physiology (Annandale, 1998). With the biomedical model, negotiation between the physician and the patient was not considered when developing a plan of care to treat and intervene with a diagnosis. The "biopsychosocial model" was coined by George L. Engle. Engle states that biological, psychological, and social factors are all involved in the causes, manifestation, course, and outcome of health and disease (Boundless, 2014). This model considers patients as the center of the care and the treatment plan. Patients have a partnership with their physician or health care provider and thus have a role in determining the path of their care. The Patient Protection and Affordable Care Act has served as an impetus for demanding patient/person-centered care. This has created a shift in how we as practitioners interact with our patients and ultimately in how we create our plan of care for them.

The use of this model is essential for successfully managing the patient/client experience both in assessing and addressing health literacy as well as wellness. The following is a patient case that will be used to demonstrate how Kleinman's explanatory model can be used to navigate and create an appropriate plan of care while simultaneously assessing health literacy.

PATIENT CASE INFORMATION USING THE PATIENT/CLIENT MANAGEMENT MODEL

Description of Patient

The patient is a 72-year-old male who is seen for complaints of right shoulder pain and stiffness. He is seen as an outpatient in an urban health care clinic. He lists his problems as follows (American Physical Therapy Association [APTA], 1999):

1. Pain in his right arm with reaching overhead
2. Limited motion with right shoulder
3. Intermittent loss of balance
4. Fear of falling especially during the winter with icy weather

Past Medical History (PMHx)

1. History of a stroke but patient is unable to give details of the type of stroke or anatomical location and so on. This occurred 4 years ago.
2. History of a fall 2 years ago with a resulting right humeral fracture that was nondisplaced, no surgery.
3. History of "abnormal heart beat" (as reported per the patient). Patient states that he has a cardiologist and that the cardiologist was recommending stents but the patient states that he is "not ready to do that yet."

Past Surgical History: None

Medications

1. Lisinopril
2. Atenolol
3. Naprosyn as needed for shoulder joint pain
4. Lovastatin

Family History

Unavailable, patient was adopted and does not know his family history.

Social History

The patient lives alone in a two-story house. He inherited the house from his mother. He has lived there since he retired at age 65 after working 30 years as an environmental engineer for the zoo that is located in the city where he lives. He has a girlfriend whom he sees every day but they do not live together. He has 14 stairs that he ascends and descends to get to his bedroom. His laundry area is in the basement and he has 10 stairs to negotiate to get to the basement. He states that he is independent with all his activities of daily living (ADLs) and self-care.

Activities and Participation

The patient is an amateur photographer. He enjoys taking photographs especially those that involve nature. He loves to travel and goes on at least three trips each year with his girlfriend.

He states that he fractured his humerus while he was taking a picture on frozen Lake Erie during the winter. He walked out on a slippery spot and was unable to recover his balance and fell.

Examination

- Posture: Forward head, loss of cervical lordosis, rounded shoulders, loss of lumbar lordosis
- Range of motion: WNLs all joints except right shoulder 120° flexion, 105° abduction, 60° external rotation
- Strength: Grossly normal except right mid deltoid and right supraspinatus, 4 out of 5 and abdominals 3 out of 5
- Function: Independent with all transfers and mobility, however, has difficulty with moving floor to stand without holding on to a chair or immovable object. He is unable to pull himself to stand without using assist
- Balance: Unable to stand unilateral stance right lower extremity (RLE) for any amount of time. Left lower extremity (LLE) able to hold 3 seconds safely. Unable to stand with close stance with eyes closed without losing balance. Unable to maintain tandem stance with RLE as dominant leg. Able to hold only 3 seconds with LLE as dominant stance leg in tandem

- Outcome measures: Timed up & go (TUG) score: 13 seconds
- Berg score: 50/56, Dynamic gait index: 18/24, Chair stand test: 10 in 30 seconds. Norm for 70- to 74-year-old male is greater than 12 in 30 seconds

Movement Diagnosis

Chronic shoulder range of motion limitation post-nondisplaced humeral fracture. Some limitation in his range of motion but overall he is able to use his shoulder and arm functionally. The patient has limitation in his balance and mobility as noted by his dynamic gait index score (DGI score). He falls into the category of "moderate risk for fall" as based on his numeric score.

Prognosis

Fair to good. Patient has a chronic condition of shoulder limitation that is restricted by chronic changes in his shoulder joint. He also does not seem to have awareness of the serious balance issues that he has or the effect of his cardiovascular history on his overall health condition. He does not verbalize any concern about his balance or gait issues.

Patient Goals

1. Ability to use right shoulder for overhead reach
2. Ability to move shoulder through the full range of motion
3. Increased strength at right shoulder as it is his dominant arm
4. Ability to use his arm to take photographs

Therapist Goals

1. Ability for patient to use his arm overhead for all ADLs safely without pain
2. Increased DGI score from 18/24 to 22/24 in 6 weeks
3. Increase ability to stand in tandem stance from 3 to 10 seconds in 6 weeks
4. Increase patient's chair stand test ability to greater than 12 times in 6 weeks

Recommended Interventions/Plan of Care

Patient will be seen one to two times per week for the following interventions:

1. Balance and gait training
2. Neuromuscular re-education for core stabilizers and right shoulder stabilizers
3. Joint mobilization for right shoulder, inferior, lateral, and anterior glides
4. Vestibular training will focus on emphasizing training beginning with eyes open and stable surfaces progressing to eyes closed as well as challenging surfaces
5. Further assessment of fear avoidance behaviors using a reliable and valid outcome measure

REVIEW OF PATIENT CASE STUDY

The model that is used uniformly in the physical therapy profession to evaluate and treat patient/clients is called "The Patient Client Management Model" (see Figure 4.1). It includes the following five aspects:

1. Examination
2. Evaluation
3. Diagnosis
4. Prognosis
5. Intervention

This model integrates quantifiable measurement, as well as history taking and mutual goal setting between therapist and patient. It also emphasizes a focus on maintaining open lines of communication. It attempts to integrate the biopsychosocial model of care. A case could be made that, without the use of Kleinman's eight explanatory model questions, a well-intentioned therapist could miss this patient's true understanding of his condition and health problems.

This patient came to the clinic truly believing that his only problem was his shoulder impairment. He realized that he could not use his shoulder and his arm in the way that he had in the past. This troubled him as he loved amateur photography and it was difficult for him to

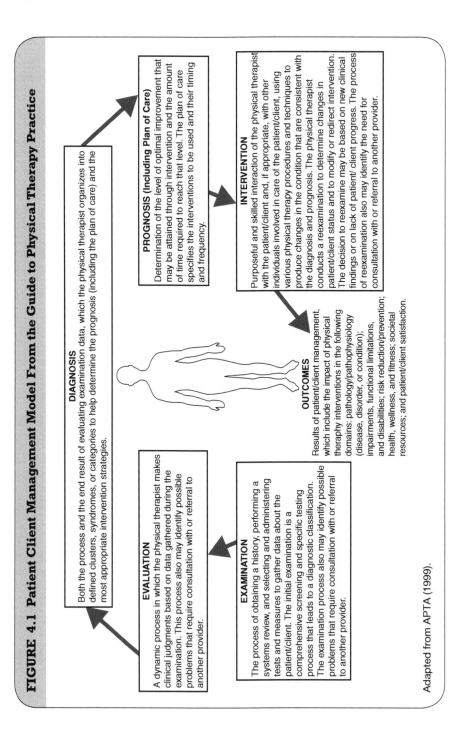

FIGURE 4.1 Patient Client Management Model From the Guide to Physical Therapy Practice

DIAGNOSIS

Both the process and the end result of evaluating examination data, which the physical therapist organizes into defined clusters, syndromes, or categories to help determine the prognosis (including the plan of care) and the most appropriate intervention strategies.

PROGNOSIS (Including Plan of Care)

Determination of the level of optimal improvement that may be attained through intervention and the amount of time required to reach that level. The plan of care specifies the interventions to be used and their timing and frequency.

INTERVENTION

Purposeful and skilled interaction of the physical therapist with the patient/client and, if appropriate, with other individuals involved in care of the patient/client, using various physical therapy procedures and techniques to produce changes in the condition that are consistent with the diagnosis and prognosis. The physical therapist conducts a reexamination to determine changes in patient/client status and to modify or redirect intervention. The decision to reexamine may be based on new clinical findings or on lack of patient/ client progress. The process of reexamination also may identify the need for consultation with or referral to another provider.

OUTCOMES

Results of patient/client management, which include the impact of physical theraphy interventions in the following domains: pathology/pathophysiology (disease, disorder, or condition); impairments, functional limitations, and disabilities; risk reduction/prevention; health, wellness, and fitness; societal resources; and patient/client satisfaction.

EVALUATION

A dynamic process in which the physical therapist makes clinical judgments based on data gathered during the examination. This process also may identify possible problems that require consultation with or referral to another provider.

EXAMINATION

The process of obtaining a history, performing a systems review, and selecting and administering tests and measures to gather data about the patient/client. The initial examination is a comprehensive screening and specific testing process that leads to a diagnostic classification. The examination process also may identify possible problems that require consultation with or referral to another provider.

Adapted from APTA (1999).

hold his camera and get the photographic shots that he wanted. He didn't understand that he still had impairments from his past stroke that were affecting his balance and his everyday activities. His health literacy regarding the implications of poststroke impairment was lacking. While using the primary care case management (PCCM), the therapist would not have ascertained that the patient did not have an understanding of how his stroke had affected not only his physical status, but also his quality of life. It is evident that the therapist who collected this data was focusing on a biomedical model. The focus of the therapist's goals was clearly addressing impairments and was not necessarily focused on the patient's whole person. With further conversation and coreflection, the therapist and patient were able to create more mutually developed goals.

The Kleinman questions #1, #3, #5, and #8 were the most revealing in terms of understanding this patient's thought processes. Of note, his fear of falling was the most limiting factor in his day-to-day life. This had created intense fear avoidance behaviors in both his home setting and social settings. He limited his activities based on his fear of falling. With further reflection, the patient was able to understand that his balance impairment was the original cause of his fall that resulted in his humeral fracture. Once these questions and fears were addressed, the plan of care and interventions took on a much more meaningful direction.

This example demonstrates how the Kleinman explanatory model and eight questions can have meaningful impact in directing a positive treatment plan. It can also be used as a tool to help practitioners assess the health literacy of a patient/client. The onus is on practitioners to assess all aspects of their patients/clients including the whole person and not just physical impairments that are noted by outcome measures.

TEACHING MOVEMENT FOR KNOWLEDGE AND SKILL TRANSLATION

Physical therapists work to teach motor behavior and psychomotor skills frequently in their practice. It is important to understand how assessing a patient's health literacy can have a huge impact in terms of choosing a methodology in which to teach patients/clients. This section will address some of the key areas that should be considered when teaching motor behavior and skill translation.

Motor Behavior

A theory that has been recognized for many years is based on the work of Fitts and Posner (1967). These authors proposed three consecutive stages in motor-learning development that included cognitive stage, associative stage, and autonomous stage (Plack & Driscoll, 2011). Each of these stages is still relevant for clinicians today when they are teaching patients/clients motor tasks. The first stage is the "cognitive" stage. If we relate this stage to our patient case example, we would find that the first few sessions during which this patient was seen would involve teaching him how to perform movements with his shoulder and upper extremity as well as movement techniques for his balance. This stage would come into play during the instruction of his HEP. The first several visits would more than likely focus on the cognitive stage. The "associative" stage is the second stage of motor learning and this involves fine tuning a skill or a movement pattern. Referring to our patient case example, we would work to help him with timing, coordination, quality of movement, pace of his activities, speed and control, in order to refine his movement patterns. The final stage, the "autonomous" stage, would come into play with our patient case example as he demonstrates ability to automatically adjust his posture, timing, and movements while he is performing a functional task such as taking a photograph with his camera while challenging his balance. As clinicians, we constantly utilize these stages during our therapeutic interactions as a guide to move forward with our plan of care. We use these stages as a way to adjust our treatment to the individual to meet the needs of his or her progression and pace. This is a helpful technique in order to respect the individual needs of the patient/client learning pace.

Mental and Physical Practice

Mental imagery (MI) and physical practice have both been shown to be effective techniques when teaching older adults motor tasks. The ability for an older adult to mentally "image" a task does not diminish with age (Malouin, Richards, & Durand, 2010). In fact, Malouin and colleagues (2010) found that vividness of MI does not change with age. The quality of the clarity of the mental imaging may be the factor that changes. They also found that the perceived vividness is what causes the strong relationship between visual and kinesthetic imagery scores for the elderly group.

Saimpont, Malouin, Tousignant, and Jackson (2013) studied the ability of older adults to utilize MI to learn new motor tasks. They did not find changes with aging when simple movements were used; however, some difficult or unusual tasks were not as clear. They also concluded that the same motor regions of the brain are recruited during MI as during movement in elderly adults. Their final conclusion was that mental practice is a viable option for older adults to learn new motor tasks and that mental practice could be used for older adults who fatigue quickly from motor practice only.

Feedback

Many authors have considered the effects of feedback on older adults while they are learning new motor tasks. Staying positive with tone of voice and with choice of verbal instructions can have a more positive outcome than negative feedback (Plack & Driscoll, 2011). Older adults are more likely than children to use extrinsic feedback instead of intrinsic feedback while learning new motor skills (Wild-Wall, Willemssen, & Falkenstein, 2008).

Special Considerations for Older Adults

In summary, there are several special considerations for older adults when a clinician is teaching new motor tasks. It is important to combine instructions for both mental and physical practice techniques. This, coupled with extra practice opportunities, will ensure that the older adult has more likelihood of success. It is also important to avoid negative feedback and enhance the older adult's ability to utilize extrinsic feedback. It is important to consider breaking down the tasks of learning a new motor activity into more manageable "chunks" to allow for greater success. Evidence tells us that adults have a tendency to become more cautious and less likely to make errors as they age (Welford, 1984).

Health Literacy Principles That Will Ensure Success

There are four major health literacy principles that will help to ensure a higher level of success for older adults. They are as follows:

1. Teach back
2. Questions
3. "Ask Me 3"
4. Motivational hooks

This section will review each of these aspects and discuss how to implement them into practice. "Teach back" is a technique in which you ask your patients/clients to show you or explain what you have just taught them. It is also known as the "show me method" and "closing the loop" (Schillinger et al., 2003). It is helpful to use phrases such as: "Can you show me what I just taught you?" "Can you demonstrate the exercises or movements that I just showed you?" "Tell me how many times a day you will do these exercises and how you will do them." "Tell me what you are going to do at home." It is important to make requests in open-ended language and in terms that the patient/client understands. It is also important to remember that you are asking these questions in order to assess how well you taught your patient/client the information and not in order to test your patient's knowledge of the information.

Questions are encouraged and sought after. Patients/clients are taught that they are in a safe environment in which there is a partnership between the practitioner and themselves. They are taught that it is natural to have an open dialogue in which questions are a normal part of the treatment. The practitioner is also encouraged to ask open-ended questions of the patients/clients. Instead of: "Do you have any questions?"; it is better to state, "What questions do you have?" This encourages patient/client reflection and not reflexive "yes" and "no" answers.

"ASK ME 3"

"Ask Me 3" is a communication technique that was developed by the Partnership for Clear Health Communication at the National Patient Safety Foundation (NPSF, 2014). It includes three simple but effective questions that can ensure that health care providers are addressing their patients/clients' concerns. The three questions are:

1. What is my main problem?
2. What do I need to do?
3. Why is it important for me to do this?

Encouraging the patient/client to ask these questions can lead to dialogue that can determine the effectiveness of treatment sessions and can lead to increased rapport and adherence with care. The patient/client can be taught the Ask Me 3 techniques from the beginning of the therapeutic relationship. This encourages increased awareness and better communication.

MOTIVATIONAL HOOKS

Motivational hooks are techniques that you can use with your patients/clients in order to generate interest and motivate them to participate. It is important to find and use something that will allow for a "connectedness" between you and them. Picking something that will focus on them as individuals that allows for their autonomy is essential. Listening to them when they describe some of their personal interests, activities, and hobbies will give clues for subjects or ideas to use as "hooks." Humor is another way in which you can create a "hook." Allowing the patient/client to feel relaxed yet involved and connected will spark an interest and maximize participation.

THE 4 "I"S

Innovative practice

Individual treatment focus

Interactive treatment

Interdisciplinary approach

The 4 "I"s take into consideration all the fundamental elements that should be addressed when working with an older adult patient. It is important to consider that each patient/client is an *individual* with unique traits and needs. *Innovative practice* is needed to connect with your patient/client in a way that will motivate him or her to engage in the partnership of a therapeutic relationship. *Interactive treatment* refers to the idea that the practitioner is not acting in a paternalistic way that uses only his or her ideas and plan of care. The partnership is mutual and the patient/client has full presence in the participation and choices of treatment. Finally, the *interdisciplinary approach* ensures that the patient/client will be treated as a whole person with the benefit of using many disciplines to address all of his or her needs.

SUMMARY

All of these techniques can be utilized to ensure that clinicians take into account the individual needs of our patients/clients. Each human being responds to, and embraces different methods to understand and learn about his or her health conditions. Once, we are able to use our clinical judgment to determine which of these techniques will fit with our clients and patients, then will we ensure success with our therapeutic relationships.

REFERENCES

American Physical Therapy Association. (1999). Guide to physical therapist practice. Retrieved from http://guidetoptpractice.apta.org

Annandale, E. (1998). The sociology of health and medicine: A critical introduction. Malden, MA: Blackwell.

Berkman, N. D., Sheridan, S. L., Donahue, K. E., Halpern, D. J., & Crotty, K. (2011). Low health literacy and health outcomes: An updated systematic review. *Annals of Internal Medicine, 155*(2), 97–107. doi:10.7326/0003-4819-155-2-201107190-00005

Billek-Sawhney, B., Reicherter, E.A., Yatta B.S., Duranko, S.G. Health literacy: Physical therapists' perspectives. The Internet Journal of Allied Health Sciences and Practice. April 2012; *10*(2):1–6.

Boundless. (2014, July 3). The biopsychosocial model of health and illness. Retrieved from https://www.boundless.com/psychology/textbooks/boundless-psychology-textbook/stress-and-health-psychology-17/models-for-positive-change-86/the-biopsychosocial-model-326-12861

Brega, A. G., Barnard, J., Mabachi, N. M., Weiss, B. D., DeWalt, D. A., Brach, C., . . . West, D. R. (2015, February). *AHRQ health literacy universal precautions toolkit* (2nd ed.). Retrieved from http://www.ahrq.gov/professionals/quality-patient-safety/quality-resources/tools/literacy-toolkit/index.html

Briggs, A. M., Jordan, J. E., O'Sullivan, P. B., Buchbinder, R., Burnett, A. F., Osborne, R. H., & Straker, L. M. (2011). Individuals with chronic low back pain have greater difficulty in engaging in positive lifestyle behaviors than those without back pain: An assessment of health literacy. *BMC Musculoskeletal Disorders, 12*(161), 1–10. doi:10.1186/1471-2474-12-161

Campbell, A.J., Robertson, M.C., Gardner, M.M., Norton, R.N., Buchner, D.M. (1999). Falls prevention over 2 years: a randomized controlled trial in women 80 years and older. Age Ageing. 28:513–518.

Courneya, K. S., Segal, R. J., Reid, R. D., Jones, L. W., Malone, S. C., Venner, P. M., . . . Wells, G. A. (2003). Three independent factors predicted adherence in a randomized controlled trial of resistance exercise training among prostate cancer survivors. *Journal of Clinical Epidemiology, 57*, 571–579.

Dossa, A., & Capitman, J. A. (2012). Implementation challenges and functional outcome predictors for elder community-based disability prevention programs. *Journal of Geriatric Physical Therapy, 35*(4), 191–199.

Ennis, K., Hawthorne, K., & Frownfelter, D. (2012). How physical therapists can strategically affect health outcomes for older adults with limited health literacy. *Journal of Geriatric Physical Therapy, 35*, 148–154. doi:10.1519/JPT.0b013e31823ae6d1

Fitts, P. M., & Posner, M. I. (1967). *Human performance.* Belmont, CA: Brooks/Cole.

Flegal, K. E., Kishiyama, S., Zajdel, D., Haas, M., & Oken, B. S. (2007). Adherence to yoga and exercise interventions in a 6-month clinical trial. *BMC Complementary Alternative Medicine, 7*(37), 1–7. doi:10.1186/1472-6882-7-37

Forkan, R., Pumper, B., Smyth, N., Wirkkala, H., Ciol, M.A., Shumway-Cook, A. Exercise adherence following physical therapy intervention in older adults with impaired balance. *Physical Therapy,* 2006; 86:401–410.

Fuentes, J., Armijo-Olvo, S., Funabashi, M., Miciak, M., Dick, B., Warren, R. S., . . . Gross, D. P. (2014). Enhanced therapeutic alliance modulates pain intensity and muscle pain sensitivity in patients with chronic low back pain: An experimental controlled study. *Physical Therapy, 94,* 477–489.

Institute for Healthcare Improvement. (n.d.). *IHI triple aim initiative.* Retrieved from http://www.ihi.org/engage/initiatives/tripleaim/Pages/default.aspx

Jensen, G. M., Lorish, C. D., & Shepard, K. F. (2002). Understanding and influencing patient receptivity to change: The patient-practitioner collaborative model. In K. F. Shepard & G. M. Jensen (Eds.), *Handbook of teaching for physical therapists* (pp. 323–350). Woburn, MA: Butterworth-Heinemann.

Kleinman, A. (1980). *Patients and healers in the context of culture: An exploration of the borderland between anthropology, medicine, and psychiatry.* Berkeley, CA: University of California Press.

Kleinman, A., Eisenberg, L., & Good, G. (1978). Culture, illness, and care: Clinical lessons from anthropologic and cross-cultural research. *Annals of Internal Medicine, 88,* 251–258.

Koh, H. K., Berwick, D. M., Clancy, C. M., Baur, C., Brach, C., Harris, L. M., & Zerhusen, E. G. (2012). New federal policy initiatives to boost health literacy can help the nation move beyond the cycle of costly "crisis care." *Health Affairs (Millwood), 31*(2), 434–443. doi:10.1377/hlthaff.2011.1169

Lascar, N., Kennedy, A., Hancock, B., Jenkins, D., Andrews, R. C., Greenfield, S., & Narendran, P. (2014). Attitudes and barriers to exercise in adults with type 1 diabetes and how best to address them: A qualitative study. *PLOS One, 9*(9), 1–10. doi:10.1371/journal.pone.0108019

Mackert, M., Donovan, E. E., Mabry, A., Guadagno, M., & Stout, P. A. (2014). Stigma and health literacy: An agenda for advancing research and practice. *American Journal of Health Behavior, 38*(5), 690–698. doi:10.5993/AJHB.38.5.6

Malouin, F., Richards, C. L., & Durand, A. (2010). Normal aging and motor imagery vividness: Implications for mental practice training in rehabilitation. *Archives of Physical Medicine and Rehabilitation, 91*(7), 1122–1127. doi:10.1016/j.apmr.2010.03.007

Martin, K. A., & Sinden, A. R. (2001). Who will stay and who will go? A review of older adults' adherence to randomized controlled trials of exercise. *Journal of Aging Physical Activity, 9,* 91–114.

National Patient Safety Foundation. (2014). *Ask Me 3.* Retrieved from www.npsf.org/askme3

Plack, M., & Driscoll, M. (2011). *Teaching and learning in physical therapy.* New York, NY: Slack.

Rhodes, R. E., & Fiala, B. (2009). Building motivation and sustainability into the prescription and recommendations for physical activity and exercise therapy: The evidence. *Physiotherapy Theory and Practice, 25*(5–6), 424–441.

Saimpont, A., Malouin, F., Tousignant, B., & Jackson, P. L. (2013). Motor imagery and aging. *Journal of Motor Behavior, 45*(1), 21–28. doi:10.1080/00222895.2012.740098

Schillinger, D., Piette, J., Grumbach, K., Wang, F., Wilson, C., Daher, C., . . . Bindman, A. B. (2003). Closing the loop: Physician communication with diabetic patients who have low health literacy. *Archives of Internal Medicine, 163*(1), 83–90.

Serper, M., Patzer, R. E., Curtis, L. M., Smith, S. G., O'Conor, R., Baker, D. W., & Wolf, M. S. (2014). Health literacy, cognitive ability, and functional health status among older adults. *Health Services Research, 49*(4), 1249–1267. doi:10.1111/1475-6773.12154

Sjosten, N. M., Salonoja, M., Piirtola, M., Vahlberg, T. J., Isoaho, R., Hyttinen, H. K., . . . Kivela, S. L. (2007). A multifactorial fall prevention programme in the community-dwelling aged: Predictors of adherence. *European Journal of Public Health, 17*(5), 464–470. doi:10.1093/eurpub/ckl272

Smith, S. G., O'Conor, R., Curtis, L. M., Waite, K., Deary, I. J., Paasche-Orlow, M., & Wolf, M. S. (2015). Low health literacy predicts decline in physical function among older adults: Findings from the LitCog cohort study. *Journal of Epidemiology and Community Health, 69*(5), 474–480. doi:10.1136/jech-2014-204915

Welford, A. T. (1984). Between bodily changes and performance: Some possible reasons for slowing with age. *Experimental Aging Research, 10*, 73–88. doi:10.1080/0144929X.2012.692100

Wild-Wall, N., Willemssen, R., & Falkenstein, M. (2008). Feedback-related processes during a time-production task in young and older adults. *Clinical Neurophysiology, 120*, 407–413. doi:10.1016/j.clinph.2008.11.007

CHAPTER 5

Public Health Perspectives on Health Literacy

TAKASHI YAMASHITA, DARREN LIU, ERICK B. LÓPEZ, JENNIFER M. STEVENS, AND J. SCOTT BROWN

This chapter provides a brief introduction as to what constitutes public health and how health literacy fits into the public health domain. This chapter also presents selected population-level risk factors related to limited health literacy by using an epidemiological approach (described later in this chapter). Particular attention is paid to older populations. This chapter concludes with a brief discussion regarding potential contributions of public health to the field of health literacy, and challenges for future research and practice.

HEALTH LITERACY IN PUBLIC HEALTH

What Is Public Health?

The most commonly used definition of "public health" is "The science and the art of preventing disease, prolonging life, and promoting physical health and efficiency through organized community for the sanitation of the environment, the control of community infections, the education of the individual in principles of personal hygiene, the organization of medical, and nursing services for the early diagnosis and preventive treatment of disease, and the development of the social machinery which will ensure to every individual in the community a standard of living adequate for the maintenance of health" (Winslow, 1920, p. 30). The mission of public health is "the fulfillment of society's interest in assuring the conditions in which people can be healthy" (Institute of Medicine, 1988, p. 40). The roles/strategies of public health are often summarized in the five Ps: (a) prevention (e.g., ill-health), (b) promotion (e.g., health education),

(c) protection (e.g., food safety), (d) population based (e.g., all members of society), and (e) preparedness (e.g., natural disasters, bioterrorism; U.S. Department of Health and Human Services, 2012).

To achieve the mission, several key characteristics of public health should be noted. To begin with, the entire population, or all members of society rather than small numbers of particular individuals (e.g., patients), are the target in public health. As the former surgeon general C. Everett Koop eloquently stated, "Health care is vital to all of us some of the time, but public health is vital to all of us all of the time." Also, public health places greater emphasis on proactive efforts to prevent ill-health of the population. This is especially different from, for example, clinical medicine, which reactively treats individuals already in need of care. Moreover, public health research and practice often employ interdisciplinary approaches integrating the science of clinical medicine, biomedicine, epidemiology, environmental science, nursing, and statistics (Winslow, 1920). Improving population health is a complex task as the nation's public health goals, found in "Healthy People 2020," includes 28 main areas of interests such as health education, environmental health, health communication, health care access, and infectious disease prevention (e.g., immunization), to name only a few (U.S. Department of Health and Human Services, 2015).

Public Health Literacy

"Health literacy" is defined as "the degree to which individuals have the capacity to obtain, process, and understand basic health information and services needed to make appropriate health decisions" (Ratzan & Parker, 2000). Health literacy plays a critical role in achieving public health goals because it enables the public to maximize the benefits from public health domains such as health education, promotion, and communication (Nutbeam, 2000). In accordance with the growing awareness of health literacy in population health during recent years, the concept of health literacy has been expanded to fit into the public health context—public health literacy is "the degree to which individuals and groups can obtain, process, understand, evaluate, and act on information needed to make public health decisions that benefit the community" (Freedman et al., 2009, p. 448). Here, the stronger emphasis is on the collective health benefits as a community and a society at large than on individual health outcomes. Additionally, public health literacy advocates for environmental health (e.g., air pollution, crime, healthy food access) through effective public health communication above and beyond individual health literacy (Gazmararian, Curran,

Parker, Bernhardt, & DeBuono, 2005). For example, effective public health communication through social marketing and entertainment education (e.g., humorous media messages to increase audiences' knowledge) can raise awareness of food environment and dietary choices in relation to type 2 diabetes among all young adults, and ultimately prevent more diseases in the community regardless of socioeconomic background and health literacy skills (Rogers et al., 2014).

EPIDEMIOLOGY OF HEALTH LITERACY

Epidemiology is one of the most critical components of public health. Epidemiological studies are designed to understand the distributions (i.e., descriptive) and causes (e.g., analytical) of ill-health as well as health risk/promoting factors in human populations (Rossignol, 2007). One of the main epidemiological approaches is comparative analysis; this approach helps identify specific populations at risk of ill-health and ultimately reveal the causes of ill-health. The association between health literacy and health outcomes has been established (Berkman, Sheridan, Donahue, Halpern, & Viera, Crotty, Vieswanathan, 2011). Limited health literacy is associated with higher risk of mortality and morbidity, more emergency room visits, and hospitalizations (Agency for Healthcare Research and Quality, 2010). Interestingly, older adults are of particular concern as they are at higher risk of limited health literacy (Kobayashi, Wardle, Wolf, & von Wagner, 2014). Also, older adults use medical services due to the combination of greater morbidity and limited health literacy more often than younger populations (Williams et al., 1995). Furthermore, older adults are more likely to misinterpret prescription medication instructions and/or warnings despite their higher usage when compared to younger adults (Weiss, 2007).

In this section, the epidemiological approach known as "descriptive epidemiology" is employed to compare the distributions and patterns of health literacy skills within the U.S. population. The older adult population is the primary focus, but other age groups are also taken into account for comparative purposes.

SOURCES OF POPULATION DATA

Most previous studies on limited health literacy used multiple assessment tools such as the Test of Functional Health Literacy in Adults (TOFHLA; Baker, Williams, Parker, Gazmararian, & Nurss, 1999) and the Rapid Estimate of Adult Literacy in Medicine (REALM; Davis et al., 1993). However, they were not collected at the population level and do not use the same standards, which creates a generalizability issue when making comparisons for public health purposes. In this chapter, we use two population-level datasets to demonstrate the importance of health literacy.

The National Assessment of Adult Literacy

The 2003 National Assessment of Adult Literacy (NAAL) by the U.S. Department of Education (White & Dillow, 2005) is a national assessment of general literacy and health literacy, which uses a nationally represent-ative sample of 19,000 U.S. adults age 16 and older in communities and prisons (Kutner, Greenberg, Jin, & Paulsen, 2006). The data collected in NAAL includes general literacy skills, derived health literacy skills, and basic demographic and socioeconomic characteristics. Although some-what dated, the NAAL is one of only a few national datasets that include a health literacy measure.

In NAAL, literacy skills are assessed using a rigorous measurement tool developed by the Educational Testing Service (ETS). Health literacy is derived from 28 health-related general literacy assessment items and then converted to a health literacy score (range: 0–500; Kutner et al., 2006). The suggested interpretations of scores are: (a) proficient (310–500), (b) inter-mediate (226–309), (c) basic (185–225), and (d) below basic (0–184). The below basic level is considered limited heath literacy. On a related note, the NAAL health literacy assessment employed sophisticated statistical techniques (e.g., item response theory) and a tailored computer program for its implementation. Interested readers may download the public-use files (i.e., data) from the NAAL website (http://nces.ed.gov/naal/) and refer to the NAAL 2003 user's guide for more details about the sampling and assessment approaches (Greenberg, Jin, & White, 2007).

The Programme for the International Assessment of Adult Competencies (PIAAC; the Organization for Economic Co-operation and Development [OECD], 2013a)

PIAAC reflects increasing recognition of the importance of read-ing, numeracy, and problem-solving skills in today's societies. It also provides information regarding international/national profiles of adult competencies (e.g., knowledge, literacy skills) as well as relevant demographic and socioeconomic characteristics. OECD collected the data from approximately 166,000 adults between the ages of 16 and 65 years old from 24 OECD countries and subregions. Unfortunately, PIAAC does not include a specific measure of heath literacy, but instead includes a measure of general literacy skills, which can be expressed as the literacy proficiency score (range: 0–500). The advantage of using PIAAC is that it makes international comparative analysis possible. Interested readers may download the public-use files from the OECD Skills Survey website (http://www.oecd.org/site/piaac/) and refer to the official report and technical guide for more detail (OECD, 2013a, 2013b).

It should be noted that, when necessary, general literacy is examined instead of health literacy in this chapter due to the limited availability of national- and international-level health literacy data. However, general literacy is a reasonable surrogate for health literacy for two reasons. First, health literacy is built upon general literacy, and therefore, individuals with poor general literacy are most likely to be health-illiterate (Kutner et al., 2006). Second, any major component of general literacy (e.g., prose, document, and quantitative) is highly correlated with health literacy (Pearson's $r = 0.94, 0.99$, and 0.89, respectively, $P < .05$) in the NAAL 2003 (Yamashita, 2011).

All summary statistics derived from the NAAL 2003 and PIAAC 2012 are weighted, and hence, nationally/internationally representative. For the NAAL 2003 data, AM Statistical Software beta version 0.06.00 was used to account for the complex sampling designs (Cohen et al., 2003). For the PIAAC 2012 data, the PIAAC online data explorer (available at https://piaacdataexplorer.oecd.org/ide/idepiaac) was used to compute descriptive statistics. These applications are available to the public free of charge. All figures are created using the statistical package R version 3.0.1 (R Core Team, 2013).

Overall Trends in the United States

According to the NAAL 2003, about 36% of U.S. adults had basic or below basic health literacy skills (Kutner et al., 2006), although the majority of U.S. adults had intermediate or proficient heath literacy. That is to say, one in three U.S. adults may not be able to perform critical health-related tasks due to limited health literacy skills. Such tasks may include administering proper medication use, determining whether and when to get vaccinated, and developing plans for personal health management (e.g., healthy weight, physical activity), which require at least intermediate health literacy skills. Given the known health benefits, the high prevalence of limited health literacy made a tremendous impact on population health and national health care costs (i.e., up to $238 billion, see Vernon, Trujillo, Rosenbaum, & DeBuono, 2007). As shown in "Healthy People 2020," improving U.S. adults' health literacy is one of the urgent public health goals in the United States (U.S. Department of Health and Human Services, 2015).

The United States in the Global Community

How is health literacy of U.S. adults compared to other economically developed nations? To make international comparisons, general literacy from the PIAAC 2012 is examined because health literacy is not available in this dataset. Figure 5.1 shows the average literacy proficiency score from selected OECD countries in 2012. The average U.S. literacy score is significantly lower than the OECD average (270 vs. 273; $P < .05$). The lower

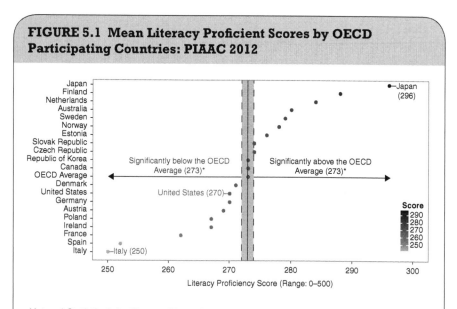

FIGURE 5.1 Mean Literacy Proficient Scores by OECD Participating Countries: PIAAC 2012

Notes: * Statistical significance ($P < .05$); between the dotted lines (gray area) indicates nonsignificant differences; data are adjusted with the sampling weights to derive nationally representative figures; OECD, Organizations for Economic Co-operation and Development; PIAAC, Programme for International Adult Assessment of Competency.

literacy score can be a serious concern in the United States considering the widely known associations between health/general literacy and health outcomes such as mortality, morbidity, preventive care, and health care service utilizations (see Berkman et al., 2011 for an excellent review).

The United States spends about 18% of its gross domestic product (GDP), nearly $2.8 trillion, on total health expenditures (Centers for Medicare & Medicaid Services, 2014; The World Bank, 2015); both sources rank the United States as the highest among all developed nations. Additionally, the U.S. health care system is well known for being complex (e.g., insurance payment system), and therefore, it demands greater health literacy skills to navigate through the system (Nielsen-Bohlman, Panzer, & Kindig, 2004). As the U.S. population ages, lower literacy skills may increasingly impact the well-being of U.S. older adults who generally require more health information and services than the younger populations (Kobayashi et al., 2014).

Health Literacy, Demographic Characteristics, and Socioeconomic Status in the United States

AGE

As shown in Figure 5.2, on average, health literacy skills peak around ages 25 to 39, which reflects the timing of completing formal education for the majority of American adults. Notably, older adults are more likely to have lower literacy skills than any other age groups despite the fact that health and medical care are most needed in later life (Kobayashi et al., 2014). Although the precise mechanism is yet to be investigated, age-related physical and/or cognitive declines seem to be associated with lower health literacy skills from a life-course perspective (Federman, Sano, Wolf, Siu, & Halm, 2009; Ferraro & Shippee, 2009). Additionally, there is a tremendous age-based variability among older adults in terms of health status (e.g., Crimmins, Hayward, & Saito, 1994). Indeed, some subpopulations of older adults (i.e., the oldest old who are 85 years and older) are at the highest risk of health problems as well as limited health literacy (Gazmararian et al., 1999).

GENDER

As shown in Figure 5.3, in most age groups (16–18; 25–39; 40–49; 50–64), on average, women have greater health literacy scores than men. Previous studies suggest that women often acquire knowledge and familiarity about health issues and health care systems more than men do because

FIGURE 5.2 Estimated Mean Health Literacy Scores by Age Groups: NAAL 2003

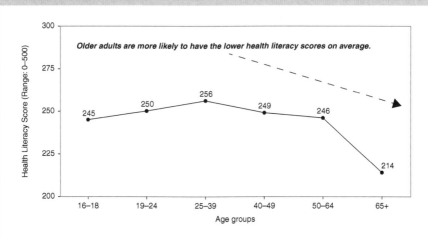

Notes: NAAL, National Assessment of Adult Literacy; Age in year is not available in NAAL; Data are adjusted with the sampling weights to derive nationally representative figures.

FIGURE 5.3 Estimated Mean Health Literacy Scores by Age Groups and Gender: NAAL 2003

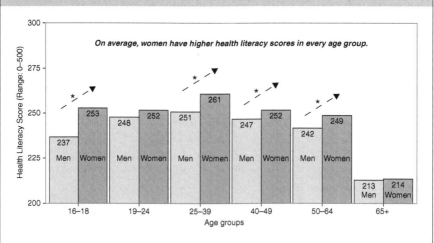

*Statistically significant difference ($P < .05$).
Note: NAAL, National Assessment of Adult Literacy; Age recorded in years; Data are adjusted with the sampling weights to derive nationally representative figures.

women, in general, face health issues more often than men (e.g., Federman et al., 2009; Lee, Lee, & Kim, 2014; National Center for Health Statistics, 2010). At the same time, health literacy skills of both men and women dramatically decline in older ages. Throughout the life course, men and women experience different health issues; therefore, gender-specific information for managing health is needed. Further research on gender differences in health literacy acquisition/maintenance over the life course would be beneficial to better understand gender inequality of health literacy skills, and ultimately health outcomes.

RACE AND ETHNICITY

Figure 5.4 depicts the health literacy disadvantages of Blacks and Hispanics in all age groups. The average scores of all ages for Whites, Blacks, Hispanics, and Other Race were 256, 217, 198, and 246, respectively. Heath literacy skills also decline in accordance with aging in all racial/ethnic groups. Public health disparities by race/ethnicity in the United States have been extensively documented over the last several decades (for an overview, see Kawachi, Daniels, & Robinson, 2005; Williams, Neighbors, & Jackson, 2003). The associations between race/ethnicity, health literacy, and health outcomes are appreciably complex. Yet, a previous national study found that health literacy functions as a mediator in the context of health disparities by race/ethnicity (Bennett, Chen, Soroui, & White, 2009). In other words, despite poorer health of racial minorities such as Blacks and Hispanics, improving health literacy may be an effective strategy to alleviate such health disadvantages.

EDUCATION

Whether younger or older, any additional formal education (i.e., educational attainment) is associated with better health literacy skills (see Figure 5.5). Educational attainment and/or years of education is one of the most powerful contributors to health literacy skills (Nutbeam, 2000; Rootman & Ronson, 2005). Arguably, throughout the life span, formal education not only improves one's literacy skills but also provides a greater number of learning opportunities (e.g., job training) as well as resources (e.g., information from highly educated peers) for further improvement. As such, higher educational attainment leads to better heath literacy skills over the life course. On a related note, education and health are closely related at the population level (Kitagawa & Hauser, 1973; Ross & Mirowsky, 1999). However, educational attainment per se may not be the best predictor of health literacy among some

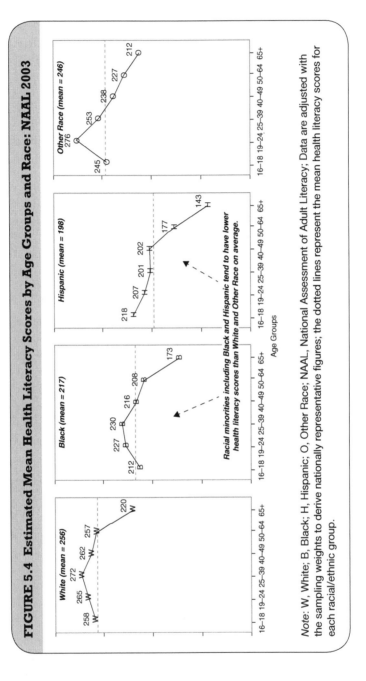

FIGURE 5.4 Estimated Mean Health Literacy Scores by Age Groups and Race: NAAL 2003

Note: W, White; B, Black; H, Hispanic; O, Other Race; NAAL, National Assessment of Adult Literacy; Data are adjusted with the sampling weights to derive nationally representative figures; the dotted lines represent the mean health literacy scores for each racial/ethnic group.

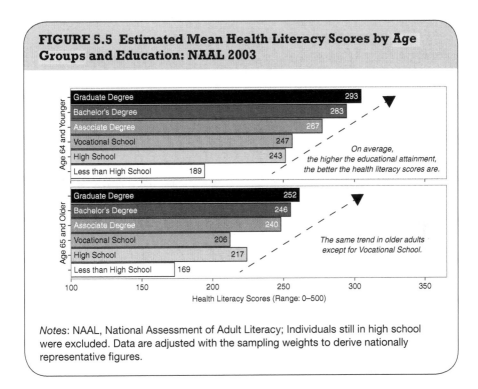

FIGURE 5.5 Estimated Mean Health Literacy Scores by Age Groups and Education: NAAL 2003

Notes: NAAL, National Assessment of Adult Literacy; Individuals still in high school were excluded. Data are adjusted with the sampling weights to derive nationally representative figures.

subpopulations such as middle-aged and older adults since their formal education often ended a few decades before. Measurement of education should be carefully chosen according to characteristics of specific-study populations and research questions (Braveman et al., 2005). Therefore, it is important to examine any learning activities and health histories in addition to formal education, and their impacts on health literacy and health outcomes, particularly for middle-aged to older adult populations.

INCOME

Higher household income levels are associated with better health literacy skills regardless of age (see Figure 5.6). Interestingly, individuals with greater educational attainment are more likely to earn higher income (Bureau of Labor Statistics, 2014). For example, the 2013 median weekly income of individuals with a professional degree was $1,714, whereas for those with only a high school diploma it was $651. As such, income levels may be a reflection of one's educational attainment, which is closely associated with health literacy skills (see Figure 5.5). It is, however, still

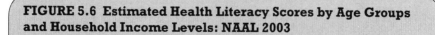

FIGURE 5.6 Estimated Health Literacy Scores by Age Groups and Household Income Levels: NAAL 2003

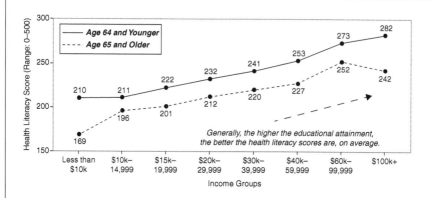

Notes: k = $1,000; NAAL, National Assessment of Adult Literacy; Individuals still in high school were excluded. Data are adjusted with the sampling weights to derive nationally representative figures.

unclear how income is related to health literacy. That is, older adults may have several other distinguishable income-related characteristics including Social Security income and health insurance (e.g., Medicare) compared to younger adult populations, and these income sources are not as directly associated with educational level as are wages (e.g., Social Security income is progressively applied, and thus, to a modest degree reduces the strength of association between prior education/working-life income and retirement income).

GEOGRAPHY

Finally, the NAAL 2003 provides limited general literacy statistics by county (National Center for Education Statistics, 2003). Using the NAAL 2003 and U.S. Census data 2000, the National Center for Education Statistics adopted a series of sophisticated statistical techniques to estimate the percentages of the lowest literacy level or "Below Basic" level for one of the general literacy domains (i.e., prose literacy: an ability to extract necessary information from continuous texts) at county- and state-level (see Mohadjer et al., 2009 for the technical details about the small area estimation). The NAAL county estimates are imported into geographic information systems to create color-coded (grey-scale) county-level maps in order to examine spatial patterns of limited literacy (The

Environmental Science Research Institute [ESRI], 2011). To identify hot/cold spots and/or clusters of counties with high/low percentages of limited literacy, the Getis-Ord Gi* statistic (Getis & Ord, 1996; Mitchell, 2005) is used and results are displayed in the thematic maps.

Figure 5.7 displays the geographic distribution of limited health literacy (the percent of adult population) at the county-level in the United States. The map enables us to visually compare and contrast nearly 3,150 counties and county-equivalent areas in the United States. The map demonstrates a tremendous variability of limited health literacy across the nation. Interestingly, the visually clear pattern of the north–south divide is observed. Results of the hot/cold spot analysis (Getis & Ord, 1996) identify clusters of counties with high-/low-risk areas (see Figure 5.8). Hot spots are observed in the southern part of

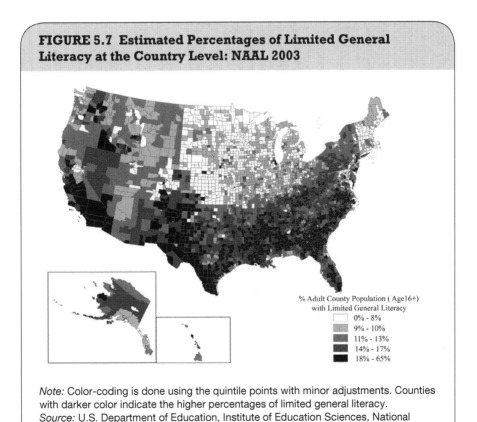

FIGURE 5.7 Estimated Percentages of Limited General Literacy at the Country Level: NAAL 2003

% Adult County Population (Age16+)
with Limited General Literacy
- 0% - 8%
- 9% - 10%
- 11% - 13%
- 14% - 17%
- 18% - 65%

Note: Color-coding is done using the quintile points with minor adjustments. Counties with darker color indicate the higher percentages of limited general literacy.
Source: U.S. Department of Education, Institute of Education Sciences, National Center for Education Statistics, 2003 National Assessment of Adult Literacy (NAAL).

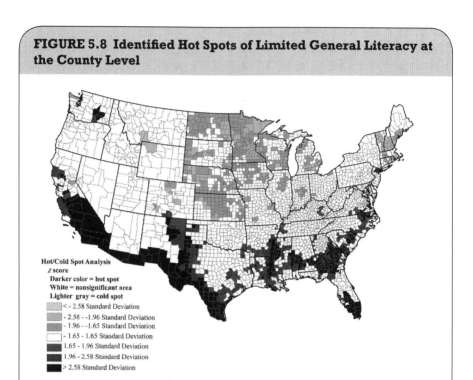

FIGURE 5.8 Identified Hot Spots of Limited General Literacy at the County Level

Hot/Cold Spot Analysis
Z score
Darker color = hot spot
White = nonsignificant area
Lighter gray = cold spot

< - 2.58 Standard Deviation
- 2.58 - -1.96 Standard Deviation
- 1.96 - -1.65 Standard Deviation
- 1.65 - 1.65 Standard Deviation
1.65 - 1.96 Standard Deviation
1.96 - 2.58 Standard Deviation
> 2.58 Standard Deviation

Z-scores 1.65, 1.96, and 2.58 correspond to 90%, 95%, and 99% of the standard normal distribution, respectively.
Note: k-nearest neighbors threshold was used for Getis & Ord Gi* statistics. Only the U.S. mainland was analyzed at county level (Hawaii and Alaska were excluded).
Source: U.S. Department of Education, Institute of Education Sciences, National Center for Education Statistics, 2003 National Assessment of Adult Literacy (NAAL).

Florida, across much of the southeastern region and across much of the southwest region (i.e., the U.S.–Mexico border areas). Speculatively, these areas have well-known limited health literacy risk factors including high percentages of older age and racial minorities (i.e., Blacks and Hispanics). However, it is also notable that another low health literacy risk factor, low-socioeconomic status, does not seem to map well to the hot/cold spots (e.g., note the near absence of hot spots in Appalachia). For many of the limited health literacy risk factors introduced in this chapter, interested readers are encouraged to compare Figure 5.8 to the color-coded maps of Census 2000 data available on the U.S. Census Bureau website (https://www.census.gov/population/

www/cen2000/atlas/index.html). For example, one might note how the percentage of Black (i.e., African Americans) and Hispanic county populations are geographically distributed in regard to limited health literacy (e.g., the hot spots).

CONCLUDING REMARKS

Contributions of Public Health in the Context of Health Literacy

As noted earlier, health literacy is relevant to key public health domains such as health education, promotion, and communication. At the same time, public health perspectives add several important insights to the field of health literacy. First, environmental factors such as community features (e.g., access to healthy food and public parks) and living environments (e.g., air pollution, high crime rate) can be added to the existing health literacy concept that focuses mainly on individuals and their behaviors (Freedman et al., 2009). The effects of the environment (e.g., neighborhood) on health behaviors and outcomes have been extensively documented (see Diez Roux, 2001; Diez Roux & Mair, 2010; Ellen, Mijanovich, & Dillman, 2001). Consideration of multilevel predictors of health outcomes and risk factors is no longer a new approach. By the same token, health literacy research should address understudied areas of environmental level (e.g., neighborhood level) influence on health literacy beyond individual characteristics.

Second, public health efforts are generally focused on large scale preventions rather than treatment of ill-health. Given that the leading causes of death in the United States are predominantly chronic diseases, which are usually incurable, a proactive approach/prevention is as important as a reactive approach or biomedical treatment/management of chronic conditions (Murphy, Xu, & Kochanek, 2013). Indeed, Nutbeam (2008) indicates that health literacy is an asset for preventing ill-health over time both in community and health care settings. Therefore, increasing health literacy may extend efforts for chronic disease preventions in addition to treatment of existing patients.

Third, in view of public health perspectives, every member of society becomes a target over the life span instead of only patients (Bennett et al., 2009; Freedman et al., 2009). Needless to say, treating individual medical cases is critical. However, the individual approach (e.g., physicians treating sick patients) does not make significant impacts on population health (Institute of Medicine Committee on Assuring the Health of the Public in the 21st Century, 2003). As such, adopting the population approach by providing intervention/information to all society members and/or high-risk groups in regard to health literacy would benefit the nation's health beyond an individual approach (Rose, Khaw, & Marmot, 2008). Hence, inclusion of health literacy in the population/public health approach could positively impact the nation's health.

Finally, public health perspectives suggest the importance of collective efforts to improve the social environment. Although individual health literacy may positively impact individual health lifestyles (e.g., proper diet, use of prevention services), social environments in communities are often overlooked. For example, individuals with limited health literacy may be severely disadvantaged when important public health-related messages about a flu epidemic, food poisoning, or air pollution need to be communicated to all members of society (Gazmararian et al., 2005). It is critical to develop a social network in communities and a public health infrastructure to deliver critical public health messages and education to every segment of the public regardless of health literacy skills (Rogers et al., 2014).

Challenges in Health Literacy Research at the Population Level

Public health perspectives have great potential in the field of health literacy. However, there are a few major challenges. To begin with, despite the rapidly growing number of health literacy studies published over the last few decades, lack of nationally representative health literacy data is evident (Gazmararian et al., 2005). The NAAL 2003 is somewhat outdated today, but it is arguably the best available national health literacy data in the United States. There are more recent national literacy data such as PIAAC 2012 (introduced earlier in this chapter), but no additional population data pertaining to health literacy has been collected since the NAAL 2003. The vast majority of influential health literacy studies have been conducted in health care settings with a relatively small number of nonrandom samples (Berkman et al., 2011; DeWalt, Berkman, Sheridan, Lohr, & Pignone, 2004). Therefore, only a limited number of population-level health literacy studies have been published to date (Rudd, 2007; Sentell & Halpin, 2006; White, Chen, & Atchison, 2008). Particularly, only a few national-level health literacy studies focusing on older adult populations have been conducted (Bennett et al., 2009; Kobayashi et al., 2014).

Additionally, a public health approach to address the high prevalence of limited health literacy is urgently needed, although a few empirically proven effective small-scale public health interventions are available in the United States (see Berkman et al., 2011 for the systematic review of existing intervention studies). A one-size-fits-all intervention approach may not be the best model due to the diversity of the U.S. population and the infamously complex U.S. health care system, (Nielsen-Bohlman et al., 2004).Providing individual interventions to all people at higher risk (e.g., older adults) is not realistic due to the high prevalence of limited health literacy and tremendous amount of required resources (e.g., funds, health literacy intervention specialists). Although a few innovative ideas such as a combination of clinical and public health approaches to health literacy (Pleasant & Kuruvilla, 2008) and the sub-population approach (i.e., targeting a unique group of individuals with a set of modifiable health literacy risk factors) (Yamashita, Bailer, & Noe, 2013) have been suggested, further discussion is needed in terms of how to address high-risk populations, particularly the older adult population (Berkman et al., 2011; Kobayashi et al., 2014).

Finally, the field of health literacy must deliver innovative educational programs to as many individuals with a high risk of limited health literacy as possible. As stated earlier, older adults are at greatest risk. Indeed, four in five older adults in the United States have one or more chronic conditions (Centers for Disease Control and Prevention, 2011). Over 20% of the U.S. population is projected to consist of older adults with multiple chronic conditions by 2050 (Administration for Community Living, 2015). The biomedical-based individual approach (e.g., one medication for one condition) to treating older adults will be unsustainable, if it is not already so. Health literacy education, which facilitates prevention of ill-health (not one specific disease) as well as chronic disease self-care, needs to be provided through public health channels (Schillinger et al., 2002; Williams, Baker, Parker, & Nurss, 1998; Yamashita & Kart, 2011). Yet, specific strategies to disseminate health literacy interventions broadly to the public have yet to be developed.

Key Messages From This Chapter

- Public health is the science and art of health promotion and prevention of ill-health at the population level.
- More than one in three or 36% of U.S. adults have basic or below-basic health literacy.

■ The average literacy skill in the United States is lower than the average found in OECD nations.

■ The known risk factors of limited health literacy include being of older age, being male, being a racial minority, having lower educational attainment, having lower income, and being from specific geographic regions (e.g., the southeastern and southwestern United States).

■ Older adults often face the double jeopardy of greater morbidity and lower health literacy skills.

■ More national data are needed to advance public health literacy research and practice.

■ The fields of public health and health literacy mutually benefit each other in improving population health in the aging U.S. society.

REFERENCES

Administration for Community Living. (2015). Administration on aging (AoA): Projected future growth of the older population. Retrieved from http://www .aoa.acl.gov/Aging_Statistics/future_growth/future_growth.aspx#age

Baker, D. W., Williams, M. V., Parker, R. M., Gazmararian, J. A., & Nurss, J. (1999). Development of a brief test to measure functional health literacy. *Patient Education and Counseling, 38*(1), 33–42. doi:10.1016/S0738-3991(98)00116-5

Bennett, I. M., Chen, J., Soroui, J. S., & White, S. (2009). The contribution of health literacy to disparities in self-rated health status and preventive health behaviors in older adults. *Annals of Family Medicine, 7*(3), 204–211. doi:10.1370/afm.940

Berkman, N. D., Sheridan, S. L., Donahue, K. E., Halpern, D. J., & Crotty, K. (2011). Low health literacy and health outcomes: An updated systematic review. *Annals of Internal Medicine, 155*(2), 97–107. doi:10.7326/0003-4819-155-2-201107190-00005

Berkman, N. D., Sheridan, S. L., Donahue, K. E., Halpern, D. J., Viera, A., Crott, K., ... Vieswanathan, M. (2011). Health literacy interventions and outcomes: An updated systematic review. *Evidence Report/Technology Assessment.* Rockville, MD: Agency for Healthcare Research and Quality.

Braveman, P. A., Cubbin, C., Egerter, S., Chideya, S., Marchi, K., Metzler, M., & Posner, S. (2005). Socioeconomic status in health research: One size does not fit all. *Journal of the American Medical Association, 294*(22), 2879–2888. doi:10.1001/jama.294.22.2879

Bureau of Labor Statistics. (2014). Earning and unemployment rates by educational attainment. Retrieved from http://www.bls.gov/emp/ep_chart_001.htm

Centers for Disease Control and Prevention. (2011). *Health aging: Helping people to live long and productive lives and enjoy a good quality of life.* Washington, DC: U.S. Department of Health and Human Services.

Centers for Medicare & Medicaid Services. (2014). NHE fact sheet. Retrieved from http://www.cms.gov/Research-Statistics-Data-and-Systems/Statistics-Trends-and-Reports/NationalHealthExpendData/NHE-Fact-Sheet.html

Cohen, J., Albright, L., Cohen, D., Hollender, D., Jiang, T., & Chan, T. (2003). *AM statistical software*. Washington, DC: American Institutes for Research.

Crimmins, E. M., Hayward, M. D., & Saito, Y. (1994). Changing mortality and morbidity rates and the health status and life expectancy of the older population. *Demography, 31*(1), 159–175. doi:10.2307/2061913

Davis, T. C., Long, S. W., Jackson, R. H., Mayeaux, E. J., George, R. B., Murphy, P. W., & Crouch, M. A. (1993). Rapid estimate of adult literacy in medicine: A shortened screening instrument. *Family medicine, 25*(6), 391–395.

DeWalt, D. A., Berkman, N. D., Sheridan, S., Lohr, K. N., & Pignone, M. P. (2004). Literacy and health outcomes. *Journal of General Internal Medicine, 19*(12), 1228–1239. doi:10.1111/j.1525-1497.2004.40153.x

Diez Roux, A. V. (2001). Investigating neighborhood and area effects on health. *American Journal of Public Health, 91*(11), 1783–1789. doi:10.2105/AJPH.91.11.1783

Diez Roux, A. V., & Mair, C. (2010). Neighborhoods and health. *Annals of the New York Academy of Sciences, 1186*(1), 125–145. doi:10.1111/j.1749-6632.2009.05333.x

Ellen, I. G., Mijanovich, T., & Dillman, K.-N. (2001). Neighborhood effects on health: Exploring the links and assessing the evidence. *Journal of Urban Affairs, 23*(3–4), 391–408. doi:10.1111/0735-2166.00096

ESRI. (2011). *ArcGIS 10*. Redlands, CA: The Environmental Science Research Institute.

Federman, A. D., Sano, M., Wolf, M. S., Siu, A. L., & Halm, E. A. (2009). Health literacy and cognitive performance in older adults. *Journal of the American Geriatrics Society, 57*(8), 1475–1480. doi:10.1111/j.1532-5415.2009.02347.x

Ferraro, K. F., & Shippee, T. P. (2009). Aging and cumulative inequality: How does inequality get under the skin? *Gerontologist, 49*(3), 333–343. doi:10.1093/geront/gnp034

Freedman, D. A., Bess, K. D., Tucker, H. A., Boyd, D. L., Tuchman, A. M., & Wallston, K. A. (2009). Public health literacy defined. *American Journal of Preventive Medicine, 36*(5), 446–451.

Gazmararian, J. A., Baker, D. W., Williams, M. V., Parker, R. M., Scott, T. L., Green, D. C., … Koplan, J. P. (1999). Health literacy among Medicare enrollees in a managed care organization. *Journal of the American Medical Association, 281*(6), 545–551. doi:10.1001/jama.281.6.545

Gazmararian, J. A., Curran, J. W., Parker, R. M., Bernhardt, J. M., & DeBuono, B. A. (2005). Public health literacy in America: An ethical imperative. *American Journal of Preventive Medicine, 28*(3), 317–322.

Getis, A., & Ord, J. K. (1996). Local spatial statistics: An overview. In P. Longley & M. Batty (Eds.), *Spatial analysis: Modeling in a GIS environment* (Vol. 374). New York, NY: Wiley.

Greenberg, E., Jin, Y., & White, S. (2007). *2003 National Assessment of Adult Literacy: Public-use data file user's guide*. Washington, DC: National Center of Education Statistics.

Institute of Medicine. (1988). *The future of public health*. Washington, DC: National Academies Press.

Institute of Medicine Committee on Assuring the Health of the Public in the 21st Century. (2003). *The future of the public's health in the 21st century*. Washington, DC: National Academies Press.

Kawachi, I., Daniels, N., & Robinson, D. E. (2005). Health disparities by race and class: Why both matter. *Health Affairs, 24*(2), 343–352.

Kitagawa, E. M., & Hauser, P. M. (1973). *Differential mortality in the United States: A study in socioeconomic epidemiology.* Cambridge, MA: Harvard University Press.

Kobayashi, L. C., Wardle, J., Wolf, M. S., & von Wagner, C. (2014). Aging and functional health literacy: A systematic review and meta-analysis. *Journals of Gerontology: Series B: Psychological Sciences and Social Sciences.* doi:10.1093/geronb/gbu161

Kutner, M., Greenberg, E., Jin, Y., & Paulsen, C. (2006). *The health literacy of America's adults: Results from the 2003 national assessment of adult literacy.* Washington, DC: U.S. Department of Education.

Lee, H. Y., Lee, J., & Kim, N. K. (2014). Gender differences in health literacy among Korean adults: Do women have a higher level of health literacy than men? *American Journal of Men's Health.* doi:10.1177/1557988314545485

Mitchell, A. (2005). *GIS analysis: Spatial measurements & statistics.* Redlands, CA: ESRI Press.

Mohadjer, L., Kalton, G., Krenzke, T., Liu, B., Van de Kerckhove, W., Li, L., … Rao, J. (2009). *National assessment of adult literacy: Indirect county and state estimates of the percentage of adults at the lowest literacy level for 1992 and 2003.* Washington, DC: U.S. Department of Education.

Murphy, S. L., Xu, J., & Kochanek, K. D. (2013). *Deaths: Final data for 2010 National vital statistics reports* (Vol. 61). Washington, DC: Centers for Disease Control and Prevention.

National Center for Education Statistics. (2003). State and county estimates of low literacy. Retrieved from http://nces.ed.gov/naal/estimates

National Center for Health Statistics. (2010). *National hospital ambulatory medical care survey: 2010 outpatient department summary tables.* Washington, DC: Centers for Disease Control and Prevention.

Nielsen-Bohlman, L., Panzer, A. M., & Kindig, D. A. (Eds.). (2004). *Health literacy: A prescription to end confusion.* Washington, DC: National Academies Press.

Nutbeam, D. (2000). Health literacy as a public health goal: A challenge for contemporary health education and communication strategies into the 21st century. *Health Promotion International, 15*(3), 259–267. doi:10.1093/heapro/15.3.259

Nutbeam, D. (2008). The evolving concept of health literacy. *Social Science & Medicine, 67*(12), 2072–2078.

OECD. (2013a). *OECD skills outlook 2013: First results from the survey of adult skills.* Paris: OECD Publishing.

OECD. (2013b). *The survey of adult skills: Reader's companion.* Paris: OECD Publishing.

Pleasant, A., & Kuruvilla, S. (2008). A tale of two health literacies: Public health and clinical approaches to health literacy. *Health Promotion International, 23*(2), 152–159.

R Core Team. (2013). R: A language and environment for statistical computing. Vienna, Austria: R Foundation for Statistical Computing. Retrieved from http://www.R-project.org

Ratzan, S. C., & Parker, R. M. (2000). Introduction. In C. R. Selden, M. Zorn, S. C. Ratzan, & R. M. Parker (Eds.), *National Library of Medicine current bibliographies in medicine: Health literacy* (pp. v–vi). Bethesda, MD: National Institutes of Health.

Rogers, E. A., Fine, S., Handley, M. A., Davis, H., Kass, J., & Schillinger, D. (2014). Development and early implementation of the bigger picture: A youth-targeted public health literacy campaign to prevent type 2 diabetes. *Journal of Health Communication, 19*(Suppl. 2), 144–160. doi:10.1080/10810730.2014.940476

Rootman, I., & Ronson, B. (2005). Literacy and health research in Canada: Where have we been and where should we go? *Canadian Journal of Public Health, 96*(2), S62–S77.

Rose, G., Khaw, K.T., & Marmot, M. (2008). *Rose's strategy of preventive medicine: The complete original text*. Oxford, UK: Oxford University Press.

Ross, C. E., & Mirowsky, J. (1999). Refining the association between education and health: The effects of quantity, credential, and selectivity. *Demography, 36*(4), 445–460. doi:10.2307/2648083

Rossignol, A. (2007). *Principles and practice of epidemiology: An engaged approach*. Boston, MA: McGraw-Hill.

Rudd, R. E. (2007). Health literacy skills of U.S. adults. *American Journal of Health Behavior, 31*(Suppl. 1), S8–S18.

Schillinger, D., Grumbach, K., Piette, J., Wang, F., Osmond, D., Daher, C., … Bindman, A. B. (2002). Association of health literacy with diabetes outcomes. *Journal of the American Medical Association, 288*(4), 475–482.

Sentell, T. L., & Halpin, H. A. (2006). Importance of adult literacy in understanding health disparities. *Journal of General Internal Medicine, 21*(8), 862–866. doi:10.1111/j.1525-1497.2006.00538.x

The World Bank. (2015). Health expenditure, total (% of GDP). Retrieved from http://data.worldbank.org/indicator/SH.XPD.TOTL.ZS/countries/1W-US?display=graph

U.S. Department of Health and Human Services. (2007). *U.S. Department of Health and Human Services Strategic Plan*. Washington, DC: Author.

U.S. Department of Health and Human Services. (2012). *Strategic plan*. Washington, DC: Author.

U.S. Department of Health and Human Services. (2015). Healthy people 2020. Retrieved from https://www.healthypeople.gov/2020/topics-objectives/topic/health-communication-and-health-information-technology

Vernon, J. A., Trujillo, A., Rosenbaum, S. J., & DeBuono, B. (2007). Low health literacy: Implications for national health policy. *Health Policy Faculty Publications* (Vol. 10). Washington, DC: Department of Health Policy, School of Public Health and Health Services, The George Washington University.

Weiss, B. D. (2007). *Health literacy and patient safety: Help patients understand* (2nd ed.). Chicago, IL: American Medical Association Foundation.

White, S., Chen, J., & Atchison, R. (2008). Relationship of preventive health practices and health literacy: A national study. *American Journal of Health Behavior, 32*(3), 227–242.

White, S., & Dillow, S. (2005). *Key concepts and features of the 2003 national assessment of adult literacy*. Washington, DC: U.S. Department of Education.

Williams, D. R., Neighbors, H. W., & Jackson, J. S. (2003). Racial/ethnic discrimination and health: Findings from community studies. *American Journal of Public Health, 93*(2), 200–208. doi:10.2105/AJPH.93.2.200

Williams, M. V., Baker, D. W., Parker, R. M., & Nurss, J. R. (1998). Relationship of functional health literacy to patients' knowledge of their chronic disease: A study of patients with hypertension and diabetes. *Archives of Internal Medicine, 158*(2), 166–172.

Williams, M. V., Parker, R. M., Baker, D. W., Parikh N. S., Pitkin K., Coates W. C., & Nurss J. R. (1995). Inadequate functional health literacy among patients at two public hospitals. *Journal of the American Medical Association, 274*(21), 1677–1682. doi:10.1001/jama.1995.03530210031026

Winslow, C.-E. A. (1920). The untilled fields of public health. *Science, 51*(1306), 23–33. doi:10.1126/science.51.1306.23

Yamashita, T. (2011). *Health literacy and health ouctomes: Implications for social determinants of health, health disparity and learning for health over the life course.* (Doctoral Dissertation), Miami University, Oxford, OH. Retrieved from https://etd.ohiolink.edu/ap/10?0::NO:10:P10_ACCESSION_NUM:miami1307717893

Yamashita, T., Bailer, A. J., & Noe, D. A. (2013). Identifying at-risk subpopulations of Canadians with limited health literacy. *Epidemiology Research International, 2013,* 10. doi:10.1155/2013/130263

Yamashita, T., & Kart, C. S. (2011). Is diabetes-specific health literacy associated with diabetes-related outcomes in older adults? *Journal of Diabetes, 3*(2), 138–146. doi: 10.1111/j.1753-0407.2011.00112.x

Fostering Independence Through Health Literacy: An Occupational Therapy Perspective

PATTI T. CALK, CAROLYN MURPHY, AND DONNA EICHHORN

Occupational therapy (OT) professionals advocate for the well-being of the clients they serve and provide instruction to their clients on self-advocacy in an effort to empower them to seek and obtain resources for their health and wellness (American Occupational Therapy Association [AOTA], 2014). Occupational therapists strive to enable their clients to access, understand, and make decisions for optimal health and participation in self-management. All health professionals must contribute to knowledge transfer by helping clients understand health information including risk, diagnosis, prognosis, and treatment options.

AGING AND LEARNING

With people living longer, the number of older adults continues to grow. It is projected that from 2014 to 2060 the older population in the United States will increase from 46 to 98 million, with the largest increase expected from 2020 to 2030 (Colby & Ortman, 2015). The growth during this decade is largely related to the aging of the baby boom generation (Colby & Ortman, 2015). Health professionals must understand and be prepared to address the special needs of older adults to empower them to take an active role in their health and well-being. Part of the process of empowerment is to address the health literacy needs of this population to ensure that older clients can access, understand, and utilize the information necessary to do this.

Being health literate requires processing of information that can be challenging for the general public, despite educational backgrounds. Aging and pathological processes cause cognitive decline that can further impact the cognitive processing required to understand health information. Trying to learn novel information can lead to frustration and anxiety in the older adult (Beier & Ackerman, 2005). It is the responsibility of the health professional to adapt educational materials to meet the special needs of the older adult. Evidence suggests that clients with low health literacy have higher health care costs due to difficulty understanding health information resulting in obtaining less preventative health care and poorer management of health (Institute of Medicine, 2004). If clients cannot understand their OT plan of care, the quality of care and treatment outcomes will suffer.

CONSIDERATIONS IN THE PROMOTION OF HEALTH LITERACY WITH OLDER ADULTS

Limited Education/Literacy Skills

Adults 65 years of age and older had the lowest average health literacy in 2003 and accounted for the largest percentage of adults with "Below Basic" levels in prose, document, and quantitative literacy (Kutner, Greenberg, & Baer, 2006). The proportion of people with inadequate health literacy continues to increase beyond 65 years of age (Gazmararian et al., 1999). Baker, Gazmararian, Sudano, and Patterson (2000) report that approximately 44% of older adults read at the lowest level (Level 1). They found a persistent association between older age and lowered functional health literacy that is likely due to age-related cognitive declines. Making inferences from health-related materials is more difficult due to these declines. Generally, clients with low levels of health literacy are less likely to ask questions and seek new information to meet their needs. Poor health literacy has been shown to lead to poor health outcomes among older adults (Mullen, 2013). It is imperative for health professionals to take the lead and initiate ways to meet the needs of these clients.

Creating learning environments in which older clients feel comfortable can be achieved by communicating respect, providing support, and linking new information to past experiences. Relating information to daily activities and typical routines will enhance learning. It is important to provide demonstration and have the individual repeat and/or practice the new skill. The more routine the new skill becomes, the more likely learning will occur (Cornett, 2006).

Culture/Demographics

While it is important to avoid stereotypes because of a person's cultural background, culture must be considered when providing a person with health information with the expectation of participation in his or her own health care management. Shaw, Heubner, Armin, Orzech, and Vivian (2009, p. 460) argued that "a person's cultural beliefs around health and illness contribute to an individual's ability to understand and act on a health care provider's instructions." For example, individuals from certain cultures may view medications as unnecessary for some conditions and would rather rely on more spiritual or emotional approaches when dealing with an illness. In addition, language barriers may result in a person's misunderstanding of health information, such as directions for medications or therapy home programs. Although a person may speak English clearly, if his or her primary language is not English, the result could be a lack of understanding of the nuances of the English language and therefore, possibly not understanding the details of the directions or health care information being provided.

Normal Age-Related Changes

In addition to the obvious outward signs of aging such as the wrinkling of skin and the graying of hair, the older adult may experience normal age-related changes in multiple body systems that must be considered. For the purpose of this section, the focus will be on those systems that would have a direct impact on health literacy.

COGNITIVE CHANGES

As a person ages, the brain undergoes some physical changes. After the age of 40 years, the brain decreases in size and weight at a rate of 5% with each passing decade (Medina, 1999; Peters, 2006). Although changes in volume can be detected through high-resolution MRI, it is not known how much impact, if any, these changes have on cognition (Medina, 1999). Research has shown that the most common areas to be affected by volume reduction related to normal aging are the prefrontal cortex, striatum, temporal lobe, and hippocampus (Peters, 2006; Terribilli et al., 2011). These areas of the brain play a role in short-term memory (STM), procedural and working memory, and long-term memory (LTM) (deJong et al., 2011; Peters, 2006; Scimeca & Badre, 2012; Terribilli et al., 2011).

These findings correlate with, and help us understand, the cognitive changes that are observed with the aging process (Terribilli et al., 2011; Peters, 2006).

MEMORY

The most commonly observed change in cognition related to normal aging is a decline in memory (Peters, 2006), but other areas of cognition such as processing speed and executive function may be affected as well (Zelinski, Dalton, & Hindin, 2011). Memory is often broadly categorized as either STM or LTM; however, memory is a complex entity that comprises multiple classifications. These multiple classifications overlap, making it difficult for the clinician to isolate one classification of memory from the next (Peters, 2006). Since possessing memory skills is necessary to learn and retain information, various types of skills, but not all, will be discussed.

Working memory, a subcomponent of STM, involves recalling from moment to moment (Gutman, 2008). This type of memory would be employed when reading instructions and then immediately attempting to carry them out. The capacity of working memory is limited in terms of the duration and the amount of information that can be stored (McBean & van Wijck, 2013).

Organizing information into usable "chunks" may aid in recalling the information (McBean & van Wijck, 2013). For example, when recalling a phone number, generally it is organized into small chunks rather than one long, continuous series of numbers (i.e., 800-867-5309). The health care practitioner may find that using the technique of chunking information into usable, easy-to-remember groups may aid the client in recalling and employing information when needed. As the client begins to recall and apply the information, it can then be organized and moved to LTM where it is stored and it becomes more easily retrieved (McBean & van Wijck, 2013).

Procedural memory involves recalling the steps of specific tasks (Gutman, 2008). For example, recalling the steps to making a cup of coffee would employ procedural memory. Repetition is necessary to encode information as procedural memory, but when it is learned, it is the most durable type of memory (McBean & van Wijck, 2013). This might be necessary when teaching clients information that will need to be used for extended periods of time. For example, when teaching diabetic clients how and when to test their glucose levels, how to administer insulin when needed, or how to manage their medication schedule, begin by providing information in various formats to be used as external cues (i.e., written, demonstration), but the client will need to practice the steps repeatedly (McBean & van Wijck, 2013). With repetition, the procedure will eventually become ingrained and can be recalled without cues or prompts from external sources.

RECALL SPEED

The speed at which information is processed slows with age and, as expected with slower processing, diminished response times to stimuli are associated with normal aging (Zelinski et al., 2011). In addition, older adults have greater difficulty attending to relevant information while filtering irrelevant information (Anstey & Low, 2004). Zelinski and colleagues (2011) point out that presenting information rapidly or using complex speech may impact the older adult's comprehension and performance.

CRYSTALLIZED AND FLUID INTELLIGENCE

Cognitive abilities can be thought of as "crystallized" intelligence or "fluid" intelligence. Crystallized intelligence encompasses knowledge that has been accumulated over the years through education, work, and life experiences (Anstey & Low, 2004). Utilizing crystallized abilities requires calling forth LTMs to employ the stored knowledge in problem-solving tasks. It is thought that crystallized intelligence increases over a person's lifetime and is less affected by aging as is fluid intelligence (Anstey & Low, 2004). Generally, crystallized abilities increase into a person's 60s or 70s, with decline evident only in late old age (Christensen, 2001).

Fluid intelligence encompasses the ability to think, reason, and problem solve in novel situations in a timely manner (Anstey & Low, 2004). It is believed that this type of intelligence is innate, and is not greatly influenced by the level of education (Stoner, 1982). STM, specifically working memory, is required to store the information that is being manipulated and processed (Anstey & Low, 2004; Manard, Carabin, Jaspar, & Collete, 2014). As discussed earlier, STM is more likely affected by aging than LTM. For this reason, a decline in fluid intelligence may be seen in the elderly. Fluid abilities peak in the person's mid 20s and gradually decline until the person reaches the sixth decade where a more rapid decline is noted (Anstey & Low, 2004). Manard and colleagues (2014) note that a relationship exists between fluid intelligence, processing speed, and working memory.

How does this information about crystallized and fluid intelligence relate to health literacy? Understanding that fluid abilities may be more prone to decline with age, health care professionals should consider building on the crystallized knowledge and skills that clients may possess. By relating information to something familiar to the client, the client may be more likely to understand, recall, and utilize the information.

SENSORY CHANGES

VISION.   One of the most common age-related changes to vision is presbyopia. Usually beginning in the fourth decade of life, the eye loses its ability to adapt from near-to-far distances and vice versa. This loss of accommodation usually results from the inelasticity of the ocular lens and a reduction in the efficiency of the ciliary muscle. This results in the lens being unable to change shape as needed to accommodate vision at varying distances (Bottomley & Lewis, 2003). This is easily corrected with glasses, but for those clients with uncorrected presbyopia, written information should be presented in larger, darker font.

A loss of contrast sensitivity and color perception may result as the lens of the eye begins to yellow. This pigmentation can cause an older person difficulty in distinguishing between similar colors, such as blue and green, and it may disrupt figure-ground if the foreground and background colors are not distinctly contrasted (Bottomley & Lewis, 2003).

The pupil gets smaller as the eye ages and as a result more light is needed for the older adult to see well. In addition, it is more difficult to adapt to changing levels of lighting in a room or while driving (Bottomley & Lewis, 2003). Instructions and materials should be provided in a room that is well lit while ensuring that the lighting does not create a glare that could inhibit the client's ability to see and read the information.

HEARING.   As a person ages, age-related hearing loss known as presbycusis may be experienced. Presbycusis is a sensorineural hearing disorder in which sounds are received and conducted through the outer and middle ear without difficulty, but age-related changes to the inner ear or to the auditory nerve result in poor transmission of sound to the brain (Bottomley & Lewis, 2003; Christiansen & Grzybowski, 1999). Although the problem is usually associated with the inner ear, changes in the middle ear may also contribute to age-related hearing loss. Changes to the middle ear may include thickening of the tympanic membrane or the stiffening of the bones in the middle ear that conduct the sound to the inner ear (Bottomley & Lewis, 2003; Christiansen & Grzybowski, 1999). The loss is usually gradual, making it difficult for persons to realize that they have a hearing impairment (Bottomley & Lewis, 2003).

Presbycusis makes it difficult to hear the beginning and end consonant sounds of words, whereas hearing the vowel sounds is not affected. High and low pitch frequencies are also difficult to hear. When engaged in conversation with an older adult who is having difficulty hearing, our first instinct is to speak with a greater volume, but the information may be heard if it is presented at a medium frequency and at a slower rate rather than at a louder volume. Older adults may also watch the speaker's mouth for visual cues to supplement the auditory information they receive (Bottomley & Lewis, 2003).

Effects of Disease That Affect Learning

More than one-third of older adults identify chronic disorders that interfere with daily living (Glogoski & Foti, 2001). Commonly identified pathological conditions that impact communication and understanding of health information include cerebrovascular accident (stroke), brain injury, Parkinson's disease, and dementia-related disorders. There are many impairments resulting from these conditions that could interfere with health literacy (Pedretti & Early, 2001):

- Language and cognitive impairments that interfere with understanding and following directions
- Slowed/delayed processing speeds
- Inability to communicate need for assistance
- Visual-perceptual deficits
- Impulsiveness

These conditions may lead to potential safety hazards, the inability to retain and follow precautions, forgetting to take medications, and/or being unaware of limitations. OT practitioners must consider these factors when working with and educating this population.

To accommodate for impairments experienced by the older adult, Mullen (2013) suggests that health information and educational materials should use fonts of at least 12 to 14 points, have Flesch–Kincaid readability scores at grade levels 7 to 8, use fewer words (approximately 250), be supplemented by verbal instructions and visual aids, and be accompanied by demonstration. Additionally, having the clients "teach back" by explaining the information back to the health professional has been shown to reinforce comprehension (Mullen, 2013).

PERSON-ENVIRONMENT-OCCUPATION-PERFORMANCE MODEL—A HOLISTIC APPROACH

One may tend to think that being health literate is only a matter of being able to read and understand information that is provided. However, the ability to effectively understand and utilize health information requires a complex interaction of many factors related to the individual's situation. The Person-Environment-Occupation-Performance (PEOP) model in OT, as described by Christiansen and Baum (2005), is client-centered and illustrates the value of using a holistic approach when providing client care, which includes improving health literacy. The PEOP model describes how the interaction between the person (i.e., physical, psychological, and cognitive abilities), the environment (i.e., home, family, health care facility, culture, and community), and the person's occupations (activities that allow the person to participate in different roles), influences the person's performance and participation in occupation (Cole & Tufano, 2008).

For example, if a person has had a stroke and no longer has full use of one arm, the following examples of each component of the PEOP model would need to be considered when determining how to best improve the person's function:

1. **Person**—How much movement is available in the affected arm? Is the affected arm on the dominant or nondominant side? Does the person have any cognitive or perceptual deficits that may also be contributing to the difficulty the person is having? Are there psychological issues also at play?
2. **Environment**—Does the person's home have physical barriers that will affect function? Are there social or familial problems that may hinder progress? Are there factors in the person's cultural environment that would influence function?
3. **Occupation**—What are the roles that the person plays in his or her life? What activities or tasks are part of the role expectations for the person that would need to be targeted during intervention? In which leisure activities does the person choose to participate?

What physical, cognitive, and social abilities are required to perform these activities effectively?

4. **Performance**—How effectively is the person able to participate in his or her occupations? What specific areas of the tasks are presenting problems for the person? Performance is the result of the integration of the person, environment, and occupation. This may be dysfunctional or functional, depending on the circumstances.

Smith and Hudson (2012) describe how applying the PEOP model to health literacy allows individual tasks (e.g., managing medication) to be broken down into the different processing skills that are required to complete the tasks. In addition, they also discuss how using the PEOP model incorporates the importance of environmental influences when performing required tasks. In order to apply the PEOP model to the health literacy of elders, the person, environment, occupation, and performance factors must be described in a way that involves obtaining, understanding, and utilizing health information.

Examples of factors related to the elderly person that can influence health literacy may include reading level, memory, visual acuity, physical ability to manipulate materials and supplies, cultural or spiritual beliefs about health conditions, and the ability to communicate effectively. Components of a person's environment that may affect the level of understanding of health information include family and other social support systems, reimbursement processes for health care costs, economic status, physical environment, and the demands of the health system (e.g., phone call reminders for appointments). The occupational tasks contributing to effective health literacy may include taking medications as directed, managing diet and exercise to promote health, understanding family history for accurate reporting, remembering appointments, and recognizing signs and symptoms that need medical attention (Miller-Scott, 2014).

The occupational performance outcomes that result from the effective synergy of the person, the environment, and the occupations result in health promotion, self-advocacy, and health/well-being (Miller-Scott, 2014). A problem in any of the areas just mentioned has the potential to affect the person's ability to be health literate. Those working with elders to improve health literacy should consider using a holistic approach. Applying the PEOP model to health literacy with elderly clients ensures that all factors are considered when determining the best method of providing health information (Figure 6.1).

FIGURE 6.1 Miller-Scott's Adapted PEOP Model That Provides a Complete Framework Suggesting the Interaction Between the Individual, the Environment, and the Occupations Necessary to Promote the Occupation Performance of Managing Health and Health Literacy

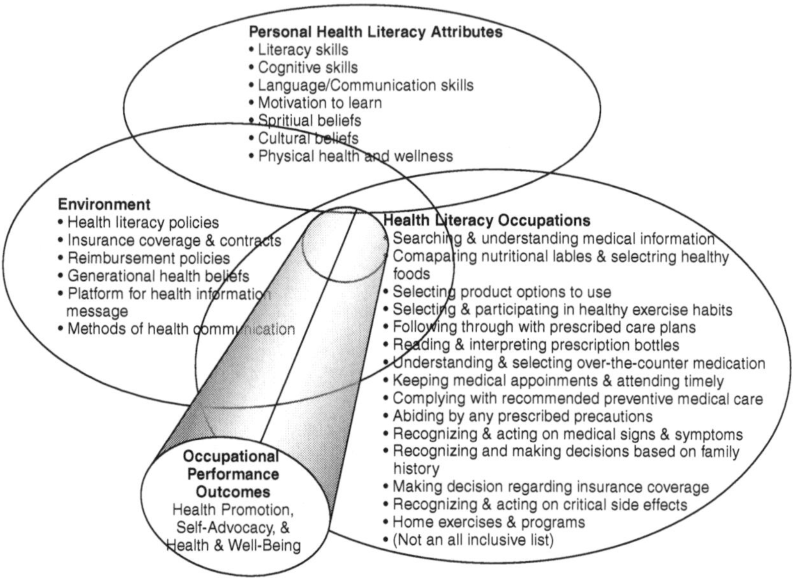

Personal Health Literacy Attributes
• Literacy skills
• Cognitive skills
• Language/Communication skills
• Motivation to learn
• Spritiual beliefs
• Cultural beliefs
• Physical health and wellness

Environment
• Health literacy policies
• Insurance coverage & contracts
• Reimbursement policies
• Generational health beliefs
• Platform for health information message
• Methods of health communication

Health Literacy Occupations
Searching & understanding medical information
Compaaring nutritional lables & selectring healthy foods
• Selecting product options to use
• Selecting & participating in healthy exercise habits
• Following through with prescribed care plans
• Reading & interpreting prescription bottles
• Understanding & selecting over-the-counter medication
• Keeping medical appoinments & attending timely
• Complying with recommended preventive medical care
• Abiding by any prescribed precautions
• Recognizing & acting on medical signs & symptoms
• Recognizing and making decisions based on family history
• Making decision regarding insurance coverage
• Recognizing & acting on critical side effects
• Home exercises & programs
• (Not an all inclusive list)

Occupational Performance Outcomes
Health Promotion, Self-Advocacy, & Health & Well-Being

Source: Miller-Scott's adapted PEOP model. Used with permission from Cheryl Miller-Scott.

PLAIN WRITING ACT OF 2010

The Plain Writing Act of 2010 requires that federal agencies use communication that the public can understand and use (PlainLanguage.gov, 2011). The Plain Language Action and Information Network (PLAIN) developed Federal Plain Language Guidelines (2011) that discusses the importance of using language that addresses the needs of individual audiences and gears language toward that particular group, rather than trying to make something meet the needs of all (Figure 6.2). It provides helpful guidelines that can be used by health professionals as they develop materials for clients written in a way that users can

FIGURE 6.2 Provides an Example of an Educational Handout Given to OT Clients That Follow These Recommendations.

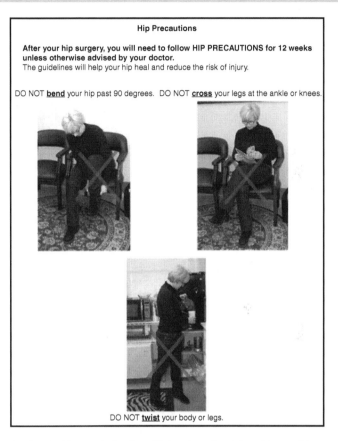

Hip Precautions

After your hip surgery, you will need to follow HIP PRECAUTIONS for 12 weeks unless otherwise advised by your doctor.
The guidelines will help your hip heal and reduce the risk of injury.

DO NOT **bend** your hip past 90 degrees. DO NOT **cross** your legs at the ankle or knees.

DO NOT **twist** your body or legs.

Source: Reprinted with permission from University of Louisiana Monroe Master of Occupational Therapy Program.

"find what they need, understand what they find; and use what they find to meet their needs" (PlainLanguage.gov, 2011, p. 2). Following PLAIN guidelines, health information should do the following:

- Use active voice
- Minimize abbreviations
- Use short, simple words, and omit unnecessary words

- Use the same term consistently for a specific thought or object
- Avoid jargon
- Use examples
- Use lists
- Use illustrations
- Explain contractions when appropriate (PlainLanguage.gov, 2011)

SUMMARY

Older adults face many challenges. As individuals age, they face physical changes in the areas of vision, hearing, muscle and joint function, skin, and hair. Cognitive declines greatly impact a person's memory, processing speed, and comprehension. Generally, health needs increase as adults age; therefore, the ability to understand and utilize health information is increasingly important. Navigating the ever-complex health care system is a daunting task that can be extremely overwhelming for the older adult.

OT practitioners aim to empower their clients to be as independent as possible in all areas of daily living including being able to make healthy lifestyle decisions. Health literacy is a key to understanding health and wellness information as well as rehabilitation plans. Creating and modifying educational materials and health care literature to meet the needs of this population by following the federal Plain Language guidelines will aid in promoting health literacy among older adults.

Applying the PEOP model to health literacy with older adults considers personal health literacy attributes, the environment in which the person engages, health literacy occupations, and occupational performance outcomes (Miller-Scott, 2014). Working together, health professionals can promote health, self-advocacy, wellness, and higher levels of independence among older adults.

REFERENCES

American Occupational Therapy Association. (2011). AOTA's societal statement on health literacy. *American Journal of Occupational Therapy, 65*(Suppl.), S78–S79. doi:10.5014/ajot.2011.65 S78

Anstey, K. J., & Low, L. F. (2004). Normal cognitive changes in aging. *Australian Family Physician, 33*(10), 783–787.

Baker, D. W., Gazmararian, J. A., Sudano, J., & Patterson, M. (2000). The association between age and health literacy among elderly persons. *Journals of Gerontology: Series B: Psychological Sciences and Social Sciences, 55B*(6), S368–S374. doi:10.1093/geronb/55.6.S368

Beier, M. E., & Ackerman, P. L. (2005). Age, ability, and the role of prior knowledge on the acquisition of new domain knowledge: Promising results in a real-world learning environment. *Psychology and Aging, 20*(2), 341–355.

Bottomley, J. M., & Lewis, C. B. (2003). *Geriatric rehabilitation: A clinical approach* (2nd ed.). Upper Saddle River, NJ: Prentice Hall.

Christensen, H. (2001). What cognitive changes can be expected with normal ageing? *Australian New Zealand Journal of Psychiatry, 35*(6), 768–775. doi:10.1046/j.1440-1614.2001.00966.x

Christiansen, C., & Baum, C. (2005). *Occupational therapy: Performance, participation, and well-being* (3rd ed.). Thorofare, NJ: Slack Incorporated.

Christiansen, J. L., & Grzybowski, J. M. (1999). *Biology of aging: An introduction to the biomedical aspects of aging.* New York, NY: McGraw Hill.

Colby, S. L., & Ortman, J. M. (2015). *Projections of the size and composition of the U.S. population: 2014 to 2060, Current Population Reports*, P25-1143. Washington, DC: U.S. Census Bureau.

Cole, M. B., & Tufano, R. (2008). *Applied theories in occupational therapy: A practical approach.* Thorofare, NJ: Slack Incorporated.

Cornett, S. (2006). *The effects of aging on health literacy.* Ohio State University College of Medicine: Area Health Education Center. Retrieved from http://medicine.osu.edu/sitetool/sites/pdfs/ahecpublic/HL_Module_Elderly.pdf

deJong, L. W., Ferrarini, L., van der Grond, J., Milles, J. R., Reiber, J. H., Westendorp, R. G., . . . van Buchem, M. A. (2011). Shape abnormalities of the striatum in Alzheimer's disease. *Journal of Alzheimer's Disease, 23*, 49–59. doi:10.3233/JAD-2010-101026

Gazmararian, J., Baker, D., Williams, M., Parker, R., Scott, T., Green, D., . . . Koplan, J. (1999). Health literacy among Medicare enrollees in a managed care organization. *Journal of the American Medical Association, 281*(6), 545–551.

Glogoski, C., & Foti, D. (2001). Special needs of the older adult. In L. Pedretti & M. Early (Eds.), *Occupational therapy: Practice skills for physical dysfunction* (5th ed.). St. Louis, MO: Mosby.

Gutman, S. A. (2008). *Quick reference neuroscience for rehabilitation professionals: The essential neurologic principles underlying rehabilitation practice* (2nd ed.). New York, NY: Slack Incorporated.

Institute of Medicine. (2004). *Health literacy: A prescription to end confusion.* Washington, DC: National Academies Press.

Kutner, M., Greenberg, E., & Baer, J. (2006). *National assessment of adult literacy: A first look at the literacy of America's adults in the 21st century.* National Center for Educational Statistics. Retrieved from http://nces.ed.gov/naal/pdf/2006470.pdf

Manard, M., Carabin, D., Jaspar, M., & Collette, F. (2014). Age-related decline in cognitive control: The role of fluid intelligence and processing speed. *BMC Neuroscience, 15*(7). doi:10.1186/1471-2202-15-7

McBean, D., & van Wijck, F. (Eds.). (2013). *Applied neuroscience for the allied health professions.* New York, NY: Elsevier.

Medina, J. J. (1999). *The clock of ages: Why we age, how we age, winding back the clock.* New York, NY: Cambridge University Press.

Miller-Scott, C. (2014). An evidence-based health literacy training program for occupational therapy professionals: Program development and evaluation. *Occupational Therapy Program Student Theses, Dissertations and Capstones.* Paper 2. Retrieved from http://nsuworks.nova.edu/hpd_ot_student_dissertations/2

Mullen, E. (2013). Health literacy challenges in the aging population. *Nursing Forum, 48*(4), 248–255. doi:10.1111/nuf.12038

Pedretti, L. W., & Early, M. B. (Eds.). (2001). *Occupational therapy: Practice skills for physical dysfunction* (5th ed.) St. Louis, MO: Mosby.

Peters, R. (2006). Ageing and the brain. *Postgraduate Medical Journal, 82,* 84–88. doi:10.1136/pgmj.2005.036665

Plainlanguage.gov. (2011). *Federal plain language guidelines.* Retrieved from http://www.plainlanguage.gov/howto/guidelines/FederalPLGuidelines/TOC.cfm

Scimeca, J. M., & Badre, D. (2012). Striatal contributions to declarative memory retrieval. *Neuron, 75*(3), 380–392. doi:10.1016/j.neuron.2012.07.014

Shaw, S. J., Huebner, C., Armin, J., Orzech, K., & Vivian, J. (2009). The role of culture in health literacy and chronic disease management. *Journal of Immigrant Minority Health, 11*(6), 460–468. doi:10.1007/s10903-08-9149-z

Smith, D., & Hudson, S. (2012). Using the person-environment-occupational performance conceptual model as an analyzing framework for health literacy. *Journal of Communication in Healthcare, 5*(1), 3–11. doi:10.1179/1753807611Y.0000000021

Stoner, S. B. (1982). Age differences in crystallized and fluid intellectual abilities. *Journal of Psychology, 110,* 7–10.

Terribilli, D., Schaufelberger, M. S., Duran, F. L., Zanetti, M. V., Curiati, P. K., Menezes, P. R., . . . Busatto, G. F. (2011). Age-related gray matter volume changes in the brain during non-elderly adulthood. *Neurobiology of Aging, 32*(2–6), 354–368. doi:10.1016/j.neurobiolaging.2009.02.008

Zelinski, E. M., Dalton, S. E., & Hindin, S. (2011). Cognitive changes in healthy older adults. *Journal of the American Society on Aging, Summer, 35*(2), 13–20.

CHAPTER 7

Explaining Radiographic Imaging to Older Adults

JENNIFER MICHAEL

The geriatric population continues to increase in number. Along with this increase comes an increase in radiologic exams performed on elderly patients. These examinations can be performed by a radiologist or by an allied health professional known as a "radiographer" or "radiologic technologist" (Frank, Long, & Smith, 2012). Elderly patients may be referred to the radiology department for a multitude of reasons. This chapter focuses on explaining the different modalities located within the radiology department and what can be expected as part of the examination process for the geriatric patient population.

PRIOR TO EXAMINATION

When being called into the radiology department, the radiologic technologist will verify the identity of the patient, oftentimes by asking the patient to provide personal identifiers such as name and date of birth. The technologist will then ensure that the physician's order that was received matches the patient's understanding of the exam to be completed. The technologist asks questions regarding patient's history to ensure the patient can perform the necessities of the exam and that there are no contraindications associated with the patient for the procedure. Patient history is taken to provide the radiologist with information that can be used to aid in the interpretation of the exam. An overview of the exam will be explained to the patient and, if necessary, the patient will be asked to change out of his or her clothes and into a gown. X-ray radiation can penetrate easily through the hospital gown material; however, denser fabrics, plastic materials, and metals can obscure the radiographic images if not properly removed prior to examination.

Some radiographic examinations require the administration of contrast agents, also referred to as "contrast media." Contrast agents are used to better differentiate between the anatomy of interest and the surrounding anatomy (Adler & Carlton, 2012). Contrast media can be introduced via a body orifice or injected intravenously. Prior to administration of contrast agents, laboratory testing to assess the body's function is performed to ensure the patient is healthy enough for contrast administration. This is accomplished through a simple blood draw.

Certain examinations of the gastrointestinal track require preparation hours or even days prior to examination. Examinations of the stomach require withholding food and water after midnight the night prior to the exam (Frank et al., 2012). The same is required for examinations of the small intestine, but beginning after the evening meal of the day prior to examination. Withholding food and water prior to these exams ensures that the stomach and small intestine are empty. Laxatives may be prescribed to patients who are constipated. It is common for patients having small intestine studies to be given instructions to eat low-residue diets during the 2 days prior to the exam. For examinations involving the small and large intestine, cleansing enemas may be administered to clear the colon.

DIAGNOSTIC RADIOGRAPHY

What Is It?

Diagnostic radiography uses x-ray radiation to visualize the internal structures of the human body. Within the diagnostic radiology department, both static images and fluoroscopy examinations are performed. These examinations are performed to diagnose and/or treat the absence or presence of a disease, anatomical structural damage or anomaly, or the presence of foreign bodies (U.S. Food and Drug Administration [FDA], 2014b). In diagnostic radiography, the x-ray beam is directed toward the anatomy of interest. The strength of the beam, the positioning of the patient, and the location at which the beam is projected is established by the radiographer (Adler & Carlton, 2012). The x-ray beam passes through the body and each x-ray photon of the beam reacts differently to the variety of materials that make up the body. The resulting x-ray beam captures the image of the body and displays it digitally or on radiographic film. Fluoroscopy examinations use the same principles but the resulting image is displayed on a live video monitor to show movement within the body (FDA, 2014a).

The Equipment

Diagnostic examinations will require the patient either to stand next to a board along a wall, sit at the end of the radiographic table, or lie upon the radiographic table. The patient's body part being examined will be positioned so that it is between the x-ray tube emitting the beam and the image receptor capturing the image. The exam being performed will determine how many images will be taken, although it is almost always more than one. Still images usually require the patient to remain still during exposure, whereas fluoroscopy often has the patient move from one position to another during exposure.

Common Examinations for Geriatric Patients

The following descriptions cover the most common examinations performed on geriatric patients within the diagnostic radiography department. Each exam has its own procedure and purpose; however, specifics of the procedure can be altered due to patient condition, physicians' orders, and so on.

CHEST EXAMINATIONS

Chest imaging is the most commonly performed exam within the radiology department. Chest images include examination of the lungs, trachea, diaphragm, heart, and aortic knob (Frank et al., 2012). Examinations of the chest can be used to verify or exclude the existence of the following pathology: atelectasis, bronchitis, chronic obstructive pulmonary disease (COPD), emphysema, pneumonia, pleural effusion, pneumothorax, pulmonary lesions, and more. Chest x-rays may also be ordered as part of the preoperative process to ensure that the heart and lungs are healthy enough for surgery. The standard chest x-ray encompasses two images taken in the upright position.

EXTREMITY EXAMINATIONS

Elderly patients are at increased risk for arthritis and bone fractures due to falls. Extremities are often examined in instances of arthritis. These studies usually include obtaining three images of the anatomy and may be taken of both the left and right sides. Examinations to assess fractures in the extremities typically include two or three images of the anatomy being examined. Common sites for extremity fractures in geriatric patients are hip, pelvis, humerus, forearm, hand, and ankle. X-ray imaging of the extremities is obtained with the patient either seated at the end of the radiographic table, standing at the upright image receptor, or lying on the radiographic table. In suspected fractures of the hip and pelvis, the radiographer will not attempt to rotate the limbs. Special imaging techniques have been developed to image the body part without having to rotate the hips or pelvis. Pathologies that may require radiographic examination of the extremities include, but are not limited to, gout, cysts, tumors, osteoarthritis, and fractures.

VERTEBRAL EXAMINATIONS

Studies of the vertebral column may be necessary in elderly patients suffering from the effects of vertebral pathologies. Examination of the vertebral column can be taken at the wall standing, or lying on the table (Frank et al., 2012). Elderly patients suffering from cervical lordosis, thoracic kyphosis, or osteoporosis can make positioning on the table difficult for the radiographer and painful for the patient. In these cases, positioning in the upright position may be more appropriate. At least two images are taken of the vertebral column for analysis. Vertebral x-ray examinations are performed to diagnose the presence or absence of the following pathologies: spondylolysis, scoliosis, osteoporosis, lordosis, kyphosis, fracture, herniated nucleus pulposus, tumor, and more.

ABDOMEN EXAMINATIONS

A variety of studies can be performed that include the anatomy of the abdomen. Abdomen examinations can range from one view to many. As part of a series a patient may have abdomen images obtained in both the upright and recumbent positions, because the contents of the abdomen shift positions as the body shifts positions. Specific parts of the abdomen require the use of contrast media for thorough examination. Studies of the abdomen are performed for analysis of the following: appendicitis, hiatal hernia, ileus, inguinal hernia, intussusception, volvulus, and more.

GASTROINTESTINAL CONTRAST STUDIES

The gastrointestinal (GI) tract does not have sufficient density to be shown through the surrounding structures (Frank et al., 2012). Because of this, contrast media is often required to properly demonstrate the GI tract during x-ray imaging. Barium sulfate is the most commonly used contrast medium utilized for GI examinations and is a water-insoluble salt mixture. Barium sulfate is not absorbed by the GI tract and is passed through the GI tract by peristalsis. When barium sulfate is contraindicated for use in an examination, iodinated contrast media is used. Iodinated contrast media is water-soluble and can be absorbed from the peritoneal cavity and excreted by the kidneys. Iodinated contrast media is used in examinations where a perforation of the GI tract is suspected. Air can also be used as a contrast agent for better visibility of the GI tract and is often used in conjunction with barium or iodinated contrast agents. Air can either be pumped into the GI tract rectally (large intestine studies) or by swallowing carbon dioxide crystals (upper GI studies).

Studies of the esophagus and stomach require the patient to swallow contrast agents during radiographic exposure. Exposures may be taken in both the upright and recumbent positions. Several mouthfuls of contrast will be swallowed during the examination and a variety of breathing maneuvers may be used to evaluate the anatomy. The patient may also be asked to rotate a full 360° to fully coat the anatomy of the stomach. Examinations of the small intestine require the patient to ingest a specified amount of barium through the mouth within a 5-minute time frame. An initial radiograph is taken upon completion of the contrast, and radiographs are then taken every 15 minutes for the first hour following ingestion. The motility of the small intestine determines how many more images are taken and how often. An average patient completes the exam within 2 hours. Patients with hypomotility can take several hours to complete the exam. The small bowel series is complete once the entire small intestine has been demonstrated by contrast media. For patients who cannot ingest the contrast media for a small bowel series, the contrast can be introduced rectally. This is accomplished by first filling the large intestine with contrast via a barium enema. Enteroclysis is another method for examination of the small intestine. Enteroclysis is accomplished by injecting the contrast directly into the duodenum through an intestinal tube. Barium enemas (BE) are performed for demonstration of the large intestine. The examination will begin with the patient lying on the examination table and barium being introduced into the large intestine through a tube that is inserted into the anus. Once the large intestine is filled with barium, air may be pumped into the large intestine as well. Patients are then given instructions to move into a number of different positions and radiographs are taken while doing so. Images may also be taken of the patient in the upright position. Patients will then go to the bathroom to evacuate the remaining barium and additional images can then be completed.

Contrast studies of the GI system vary on their scale of discomfort and length of procedure. Geriatric patients may find that swallowing the contrast media is difficult and run an increased risk for aspirating the contrast agents. The best way to minimize discomfort and the length of the procedure is to follow all preparatory and postexamination measures. Barium enemas can be particularly strenuous for elderly patients. For this reason, the radiographer will verbally consult the patient to evaluate his or her strength and alertness throughout the exam process. All examinations involving contrast media will require patients to flush their system with plenty of water for the days following the examination. This is especially important for geriatric patients whose digestive systems may already have decreased functionality. Contrast studies are performed to diagnose bowel obstruction, diverticulitis, gastroesophageal reflux, pyloric stenosis, ulcerative colitis, polyps, esophageal varices, achalasia, and more.

BONE DENSITOMETRY

What Is It?

Bone densitometry is conducted to measure the bone mineral content of the body and assess bone strength (Frank et al., 2012). Dual energy x-ray absorptiometry (DXA) is the most commonly used bone measuring technique. DXA uses low-energy ionizing radiation.

A patient's peak bone mass is reached between the ages of 20 to 30 years. In women, bone mass begins to decrease around the age of 50 and becomes more significant in postmenopausal women. In men this period of decreased bone mass begins around 65. A decrease in bone mass can result in osteoporosis. It is estimated that 10 million Americans have osteoporosis and 80% of those suffering from osteoporosis are women. When osteoporosis is present, the patient is at risk for fragility fractures. Osteoporosis is a multifactorial disease with no exact known cause; however, the following risk factors must be considered:

- Caucasian
- Increased age
- Female
- Smoker
- Low estrogen levels
- Family history

- Prior fractures as an adult
- Low body weight/low BMI

The Examination

Patients who are receiving a bone density examination will be transported to the room where the examination will take place. The patient can expect to be asked to change into a hospital gown and lie on the examination table. DXA equipment will take measurements of the patient's lower back and hip(s); there is also equipment that takes measurements of the forearm. The exam is relatively short and with minimal discomfort, usually from lying on the examination table. The densities of the areas examined are measured and averaged. The results of these measurements, combined with other diagnosing techniques, aid in the following ways:

- Assist in diagnosis of low bone density
- Assess bone strength, monitor effects of therapy on the bones
- Predict fracture risk

MAMMOGRAPHY

What Is It?

Mammography is medical imaging of the breast and its primary goal is to detect breast cancer (National Institutes of Health [NIH], 2015). Early detection of breast cancer, along with proper diagnosis and treatment, increases a patient's survival rate. Mammography can detect breast cancer before it is palpable and has become the standard screening tool for breast cancer. Typically women begin to receive mammograms between the ages of 40 and 50. A physician assesses a patient's need for a mammogram based on these risk factors (Frank et al., 2012):

- Age: The occurrence of breast cancer increases with age.
- Hormones: Hormone changes associated with pregnancy, lactation, and menopause affect the breast tissue. There is an increased risk in women who began menses before the age of 12, began menopause after the age of 52, women who never bore children, and/or had their first birth after the age of 30.

- Family History: Women who have a female relative who is closely related and had breast cancer are at an increased risk of having breast cancer themselves (i.e., sister, daughter, mother).
- Breast Cancer Genes: Two genes have been identified that are linked to breast cancer: BRCA1 and BRCA2. Men and women who are carriers of these genes are at increased risk of breast, cervical, and testicular cancers.

All women are recommended to have mammograms performed every 1 to 2 years beginning at age 50 if they have not already started screening (NIH, 2015). Women who are at high risk for breast cancer or show other symptoms of the disease may be recommended for early mammography screenings. Symptoms of breast cancer include: breast lump, nipple discharge, breast pain, breast skin dimpling, and nipple appearance changes.

The Examination

Upon entering the examination room, the patient will answer a few medical history questions and then will be asked to remove clothing from the waist up and put on a gown with an opening in the front. The patient may also be asked to remove any deodorant or antiperspirant; these substances can be mistaken as calcifications in the breast if they appear on the image. Routine screenings of the breast consist of two images being obtained. The breast is positioned atop of the x-ray plate and a compressor is moved down upon the breast to help flatten the breast tissue. In patients with very large or very dense breasts, additional views, views with magnification, or views with increased compression may be necessary to achieve a diagnostic quality image. Patients with breast implants can expect additional views to be obtained; images with and without the implant pictured are necessary. The breasts are examined one at a time and are both imaged for comparison purposes. The images are taken by a mammographer. Once the radiologist examines the images, the patient may be asked to come back for additional images to be obtained. This is quite common and simply means the radiologist wants to recheck an area that was not well visualized on the first radiographs.

RADIATION THERAPY/RADIATION ONCOLOGY

What Is It?

There are three principle modalities for treating cancer: surgery, chemotherapy, and radiation therapy (Frank et al., 2012). Radiation therapy uses high doses of radiation to kill cancer cells and to keep them from spreading. The goal of radiation treatment is to deliver a high dose of radiation specifically to the cancerous tumor, while minimizing the amount of radiation normal, noncancerous tissue receives.

The Therapy Treatment

Prior to receiving radiation therapy, the oncologist will have the patient undergo a variety of imaging exams within the radiology department to better visualize the size, location, and anatomic extent of the tumor. The next step may be to biopsy the tumor and have it examined by a pathologist. Seventy-five percent of diagnosed cancer patients undergo radiation treatment. The length of radiation treatment varies, but averages 5 days a week for 2 to 8 weeks.

Dosimetrists are consulted by the oncologist to determine the appropriate radiation dose for each specific tumor or target area. Each organ in the body has a radiation tolerance limit. Dosimetrists help determine the strength of the dose necessary to kill the cancer cells, but not result in organ failure to the affected or adjacent organs. Once the patient has completed the pretreatment exams, the oncologist will determine the treatment volume and area to receive the radiation. The treatment area includes the tumor as well as a small surrounding area that would include the draining lymphatics and surrounding tissue to account for patient movement. It is highly important that the patient remain still and in the exact position as instructed by the radiation therapist during treatment. If the patient does not follow the positioning instructions, normal tissue may be inadvertently irradiated and the tumor may not. A radiation therapist may use devices known as immobilization devices to keep the patient still during exposure.

NUCLEAR MEDICINE

What Is It?

Once described as "inside out" imaging, nuclear medicine is a way to record radiation being emitted by the patient's body (American Society of Radiologic Technologists [ASRT], 2002). Nuclear medicine uses radiopharmaceuticals (radioactive materials) to diagnose, treat, and conduct research for a variety of diseases and pathologies. Other areas within radiology diagnose the presence of disease based on structural abnormalities, whereas nuclear medicine assesses organ or tissue function. Radiopharmaceuticals, known as "tracers," can be introduced into the body by injection, inhalation, or ingestion. The tracer used depends on the specific part of the body being studied. Tracers emit gamma rays that are converted into a diagnostic image through a device known as a "gamma camera."

The Examination

There are a wide variety of tests that take place within the nuclear medicine modality. Prior to the exam, a nuclear medicine technologist will explain the procedure to the patient, answer any questions, and assist the patient throughout the procedure. The technologist will administer the radioactive material to the patient and begin obtaining images. The procedure can last minutes to hours, or even days. The exams that require imaging over a period of days will require the patient to go home after the initial images are taken and return the next day, and so on. The radiopharmaceuticals will be eliminated from the patient's body naturally; however, an increase in fluid intake can help eliminate them more quickly. The radiation dose on average for nuclear medicine exams is equal to or less than that of a standard chest x-ray. Patients may be given simple acts such as flushing the toilet twice after use to limit the amount of radiation exposure to those who share a household with the exposed individual.

COMPUTED TOMOGRAPHY

What Is It?

Computed tomography, also known as "CT," once went by the term "CAT scan." Once this imaging modality was converted from film to computer display imaging, its name also changed. The CAT (computed axial tomography) unit was the first imaging scanner that produced images that would image the body in "slices." These slices are cross-sectional images of the body. In diagnostic x-ray, the patient is positioned between the tube that emits the radiation and the image receptor that creates the image. The image results in body structures that are superimposed over one another. In CT, the x-ray tube and image receptor rotate around the patient; this imaging technique eliminates the superimposition of anatomical structures. Where diagnostic x-ray represents two-dimensional images of the body, CT represents three-dimensional imaging.

The Examination

During the examination the patient lies on a flat table that moves in and out of the CT gantry. The gantry is a circular device that allows for the x-ray tube and imaging receptor to circle the patient during examination. Upon scheduling the examination, patients will be instructed on any restrictions associated with medications or food/water intake. Prior to examination the technologist will explain the procedure to the patient, have the patient change into a hospital gown (if necessary), and answer any questions regarding the procedure. Patients will be instructed to remove any objects that are metal including eyeglasses, jewelry, dentures, or hair accessories. Patients receiving oral contrast will be instructed to drink it prior to their examination. Other patients may receive intravenous contrast during their exam, and for other patients, no contrast may be necessary.

CT provides high-resolution imaging and is the fastest and most accurate tool for exams of the abdomen, chest, and pelvis. CT examinations are completed within minutes, which makes CT imaging ideal for individuals suffering from motor vehicle accidents, acute chest or abdominal pain, or those with difficulty breathing. CT is also often used in conjunction with radiation therapy to provide the most accurate delivery of high-radiation doses to cancerous tumors. During the exam it is essential that the patient remain very still and follow the instructions of the technologists. Patients can be expected to have to hold their breath for periods of time during the exam.

Like all medical procedures, CT has its benefits and risks. The radiation dose to the patient is much higher for CT exams when compared to other radiologic examinations. Because of this, no other individuals are typically permitted in the room during the exam. The CT scan itself is painless and allows for quality examination of bone, soft tissue, organs, and blood vessels. When compared to magnetic resonance imaging (MRI), which also creates 3D cross-sectional imaging, CT is less sensitive to patient movement and allows for patients with implanted medical devices to be examined.

MAGNETIC RESONANCE IMAGING

What Is It?

Similar to CT, MRI is an imaging technique that provides cross-sectional images of the body by noninvasive measures (Frank et al., 2012). However, quite the opposite from CT, MRI does not use any ionizing radiation. Instead, MRI uses magnetic fields and radio waves to capture its images. While positioned within the MRI's magnetic field, radio waves are used to redirect the alignment of hydrogen atoms, which naturally exist in the body. This realignment of the hydrogen atoms does not cause any chemical change within the body, but as they return to their original alignment they emit an energy that can be measured by the MRI scanner; this measurement is used to create a picture of the tissue. MRI is often the best modality for imaging the differentiation between abnormal and normal tissue. Computed tomography and magnetic resonance imaging both provide cross sectional imaging of the body. However, MRI is more likely to identify pathology or diseases in soft tissue structures.

The Examination

Prior to examination the patient will be questioned regarding patient history. It is vital for an MRI technologist to be abreast of any prior surgeries a patient may have had (Radiological Society of North America [RSNA], 2014a). Patients with the following implants may not be compatible with MRI examinations:

- Cochlear implants
- Brain aneurysm clips
- Blood vessel coils
- Cardiac defibrillators / pacemakers

All patients will need to change into a hospital gown and remove any metal objects. The patient will then lie on a table and a positioning device or "coil" may be utilized and placed onto the patient for the duration of the exam. The coils make examination of superficial structures more easily obtained. Once the patient is on the table, the patient is given ear plugs or head phones to wear throughout the procedure. The MRI machine will go through a series of loud tapping or thumping sounds. Facilities utilize ear protective devices to reduce the noise of the machine. Many departments have the ability to play music for the patient through the headphones during the procedure. The table will move the patient into the magnetic field for the exam. MRI exams can be performed with or without contrast, or both. Patients who suffer from claustrophobia or anxiety may be administered a mild sedative before beginning the MRI exam. The MRI machine can be perceived as a tight space and the exams are rather lengthy; the average time for an MRI exam ranges from 30 to 50 minutes. Individuals requiring sedation account for about 5% of MRI patients. MRI exams are painless; however, patients do find it uncomfortable to remain still during the imaging process.

ULTRASONOGRAPHY

What Is It?

Another imaging modality within the radiology department that does not use ionizing radiation to obtain images of the body is ultrasound. Prenatal exams are typically the first imaging exam that individuals think of when hearing the term ultrasound, but ultrasound can be used to image the heart, blood vessels, kidney, liver, and more. Ultrasound can also be used to guide needles for biopsy procedures. Ultrasound images are obtained by emitting ultrasonic sound waves into the body and transmitting the sound waves into images as they are reflected back from the body's structures and vessels (Frank et al., 2012). A small transducer emits the sound waves and collects the reflected sound waves. This information is then converted to imagery by a computing system and displayed on an ultrasound monitor. Ultrasound not only displays the anatomy of the body but can also evaluate blood flow through vessels. Recent advancements in sonography have introduced a three-dimensional format, although most imaging is still displayed in thin, flat, two-dimensional sections of the body.

The Examination

Depending on the area being examined, the patient may be instructed to withhold ingestion of food or drink for up to 12 hours prior to the exam (RSNA, 2014b). Other procedures may require ingestion of up to six glasses of water within the 2 hours prior to examination.

Patients may or may not be instructed to empty their bladder prior to the performance of the exam. The patient's clothing will need to be removed from the area being examined; this may result in the patient having to be gowned or simply removing the clothing from the area of interest. Ultrasound gel will be applied generously to the patient's skin, and the ultrasound transducer will be placed on the gel. The majority of ultrasounds use a transducer that is placed on the outside of the body on the skin; however, there are three types of probes that can be attached to a transducer and inserted into the body. These probes are utilized in the following exams:

- Transrectal ultrasound: Utilized in exams to assess the prostate; this probe is inserted into the rectum.
- Transvaginal ultrasound: Utilized to image the uterus and ovaries; this probe is inserted vaginally.
- Transesophageal echocardiogram: Utilized to examine the heart; this probe is inserted through the esophagus.

Overall, ultrasound may result in mild discomfort, but should be painless. The average ultrasound takes 30 minutes to complete, but can range from 10 minutes to an hour depending on the extensiveness of the exam.

Ultrasound offers noninvasive, real-time imaging and poses no risk of exposure to ionizing radiation. Ultrasound is often a less-expensive option than other imaging modalities for obtaining a clear picture of soft tissue; however, ultrasound is limited in areas that are air or gas filled. The sound waves that are utilized in ultrasound are disrupted by air and gas; therefore, in patients with air-filled bowels, diagnostic radiography, CT scanning, or MRI imaging may provide better diagnostic quality.

CARDIOVASCULAR-INTERVENTIONAL RADIOLOGY

What Is It?

Procedures performed within the interventional radiology (IR) department are minimally invasive procedures that utilize radiographic imaging to diagnose and treat pathologies (Johns Hopkins Medicine, n.d.). The ability of IR to intervene in the course of a medical condition makes it a therapeutic procedure. IR is used for nearly every organ system and has less associated risk, pain, and recovery time than open surgery procedures. Physicians perform the procedures with the help of specially trained radiographers, anesthetists, and nurses. "Angiography," a radiographic examination that introduces iodinated contrast and/ or gas into the vascular structures of the body (Frank et al., 2012), is the general term for the type of examinations performed within this department. Procedures may be performed using local and/or general anesthesia.

The Equipment

Needles, guidewires, sheaths, and catheters can all be used within IR procedures along with radiographic and fluoroscopy equipment. This imaging equipment is used to guide and document other devices as they are introduced into a variety of veins, arteries, and vessels (Frank et al., 2012). Vascular access is achieved with a needle. A guidewire is then inserted into the hole of the needle. Internal needle diameter and guidewire size must be appropriately paired to each other and appropriately selected based on patient size and vessel entry. Guidewires are used as a guide for where a catheter is to be placed. Catheters are used to introduce contrast into vessels, and can also open blocked passages. The most commonly punctured vessels are the femoral, axillary, brachial, and radial arteries and/or veins. Interventional procedures are performed under sterile conditions to prevent infection.

The Examination

A thorough explanation of the procedure along with written consent from the patient is required for IR studies. Previous severe reactions to iodinated contrast media, impaired renal function, or inability to tolerate general anesthesia are all reasons a physician may determine a patient unfit for an IR procedure. Patients are usually restricted to a clear intake diet prior to the procedure and certain medications may be withheld. Patients not being administered general anesthesia will be communicated throughout the procedure by the IR team for patient reassurance and expectations, and may be administered a mild sedative prior to beginning the procedure.

Aortography is placement of a catheter within the aorta for the introduction of contrast to image the aorta with radiographic equipment

(Frank et al., 2012). Aortography is performed with the patient supine. Contrast is injected while frontal and lateral images are obtained simultaneously. Thoracic aortography is used in patients with aortic dissection; whereas abdominal aortography evaluates abdominal aortic aneurysm, occlusion, or atherosclerotic disease.

Arteriography is radiographic imaging of the arteries with the introduction of contrast media. Abdominal visceral arteriography is performed to diagnose the presence or absence of atherosclerotic disease, thrombosis, occlusion, and bleeding (Frank et al., 2012). Celiac and hepatic arteriography are performed to visualize the celiac and common hepatic arteries that carry blood to the stomach, proximal duodenum, liver, spleen, and pancreas. From the aorta arises the right and left renal arteries; renal arteriography is performed to visualize the blood supply from the aorta to the kidneys. To show anatomy and diagnose pathology within the abdomen, other arteries that branch from the aorta may also be selectively studied.

Cardiac catheterization is also a component of interventional radiography. Cardiac catheterization can be performed for diagnostic purposes to treat a condition through therapeutic measures (Frank et al., 2012). It is a minor surgical procedure that introduces specialized catheters in the heart. These catheters can be used to introduce contrast or can be used to treat a variety of cardiovascular disorders.

SUMMARY

The geriatric population is at the highest point the world has ever seen. The continuing advances in health care are expected to aid in continuing to increase this population group. The radiology department plays a large part in treating and diagnosing the ever-growing geriatric population. By explaining these complex procedures in plain language, patients can understand the techniques. Using pictures can be invaluable in aiding understanding of the procedures.

REFERENCES

Adler, A., & Carlton, R. (2012). *Introduction to radiologic sciences and patient care.* St. Louis, MO: Elsevier.

American Society of Radiologic Technologists. (2002). Nuclear medicine imaging. Retrieved from https://www.asrt.org/docs/patientpages/asrt2011_nucmed.pdf

Frank, E. D., Long, B. W., & Smith, B. J. (2012). *Merrill's atlas of radiographic positioning & procedures* (Vols. 1–3., 12th ed.). St. Louis, MO: Elsevier.

Johns Hopkins Medicine. (n.d.). *What is vascular and interventional radiology*. Retrieved from http://www.hopkinsmedicine.org/vascular/what_is_IR.html

National Institutes of Health. (2015). *Mammography*. Retrieved from http://www.nlm.nih.gov/medlineplus/ency/article/003380.htm

Radiological Society of North America. (2014a). Magnetic resonance imaging (MRI)—Body. Retrieved from http://www.radiologyinfo.org/en/info.cfm?pg=bodymr

Radiological Society of North America. (2014b). Ultrasound—General. Retrieved from http://www.radiologyinfo.org/en/info.cfm?pg=genus

U.S. Food and Drug Administration (FDA). (2014a). Fluoroscopy. Retrieved from http://www.fda.gov/Radiation-EmittingProducts/RadiationEmittingProducts andProcedures/MedicalImaging/MedicalX-Rays/ucm115354.htm

U.S. Food and Drug Administration (FDA). (2014b). Radiography. Retrieved from http://www.fda.gov/Radiation-EmittingProducts/RadiationEmittingProducts andProcedures/MedicalImaging/MedicalX-Rays/ucm175028.htm

CHAPTER 8

Helping Older Adults Understand Medication and Treatment Regimens

LORI M. METZGER

Understanding health literacy in the presence of medication management and treatment regimens is a unique and vital piece to successful self-management of health care needs. Each one of us wants to be independent in caring for ourselves and demonstrate self-efficacy, that is, believing that one can perform self-care behaviors even under varying conditions (Chia, Schlenk, & Dunbar-Jacob, 2006). As we grow older, self-care may become more challenging but is still certainly possible, given we have the appropriate tools. The skill of health literacy is crucial to navigating health care needs for older adults. Health literacy is key to health promotion and thereby affects the well-being of each one of us (Zamora & Clingerman, 2011). When a client is not able to understand the instructions of the health care provider, he or she will not be able to follow the instructions placing the client's health care in jeopardy.

Poor health literacy has long been linked with adverse health outcomes in older adults (Agency for Healthcare Quality and Research [AHRQ], 2015a). Understanding health care treatments, client education, and written instructions are key to managing chronic health conditions and thereby preventing poor health outcomes. Perhaps the most important health education and clear understanding for older adults to possess is that of medications. Knowing that older adults are prescribed more medications than any other age group, it is estimated that 80% of persons over the age of 65 have at least one chronic disease and 68% manage two chronic diseases (National Council on Aging [NCOA], 2015). Older adults average 5.7 medications in order to manage chronic diseases (Sirey, Greenfield, Weinberger, & Bruce, 2013). For many older adults, the ability to remain independent and in their home depends on the ability to manage chronic disease. Being able to read and understand interventions that assist older adults in managing their medications and treatments can help to prevent these adverse health outcomes and will subsequently improve their quality of life. Thus, this begs the question, how can health care professionals overcome health literacy in older adults to avoid negative outcomes?

MEDICATION ADHERENCE

First, let's explore the importance of medication compliance or adherence. The term "medication compliance" has fallen out of use and the newer term of "medication adherence" is now consistently used in the literature. Medication compliance is defined as the process of complying to a demand or proposal and implies coercion. Compliance infers a one-way relationship of the health care provider giving instruction with little participation of the client (MacLaughlin et al., 2005). The term adherence implies an action on the part of the client or patient rather than implying blame as does the word compliance. Adherence also infers a collaborative versus a passive role on the part of the client (Haugh, 2014; MacLaughlin, et al., 2005). A dialogue or two-way communication is essential for the client's effective understanding of health care instruction and the term adherence indicates that there is an active role for both the health care provider and client. Medication adherence is best achieved when there is an effective partnership between the health care provider and client (MacLaughlin et al., 2005).

Adhering or "sticking to" a medical or treatment regimen is important in assisting the client to achieve goals, prevent disease progression, and avoid adverse events, even a higher risk of mortality (Zhang, Terry, & McHorney, 2014). Adhering to a plan of care, or list of medications, is especially challenging when the client doesn't understand *how* to do so. Nonadherence impedes the client's ability to achieve health goals but is also considered a serious threat to the economic health of the United States (Jones, Treiber, & Jones, 2014). In the United States, the cost of poor medication adherence is estimated to cost $100 billion for excess hospitalizations and up to an estimated $290 billion *per year* in health care costs that are very possibly preventable. The financial impact of nonadherence is overwhelming (Jones et al., 2014).

Understanding the many reasons for medication nonadherence helps health care providers in removing barriers and improving not only the understanding of medication and treatment regimens but health outcomes as well. Effectively managing medications and treatment regimens is a multifactorial process that needs to be highly individualized.

Not all factors can be controlled, such as age of the client, memory issues, or ethnicity. However, health literacy is a factor on which health care professionals can and should have an impact. While there is conflicting evidence regarding a definite association between health literacy and medication in older adults, there is no doubt that clients with adequate health literacy are much better equipped to manage chronic disease states than those with low health literacy (Bauer et al., 2013; Loke, Hinz, Wang, & Salter, 2012).

BARRIERS TO MEDICATION ADHERENCE

Some barriers to following medication and treatment regimens are fixed and the health care providers can have no impact. These include age, race, ethnicity, and some researchers would posit that even gender is a barrier to medication adherence (Holt et al., 2013). Holt and colleagues (2013) have found that women with chronic depression had a higher association with nonadherence than men. This appears to be the only concrete evidence in the literature relative to gender. It is obvious that these barriers are nonmodifiable, but as we move into cultural beliefs and personality, it is possible to educate the client based on factual evidence that medications and treatments can and do work. The ethnicity or cultural beliefs of a client can heavily influence how a client views or respects the health care provider, especially the physician or nurse practitioner providing the prescription. How a client perceives health, a negative or positive attitude, and personality is a difficult aspect to alter but should be considered a modifiable factor. Sirey and colleagues (2013) have found that positive attitudes or perceived need are predictive of treatment adherence and effective client participation. Additionally, negative attitudes, such as stigma or myths about care, were also predictive relative to adherence of a plan of care (Sirey, Bruce, & Alexopoulos, 2001). Certainly, an individual's underlying definition or philosophy of health lifestyle is related to not only medication adherence but self-efficacy (Holt et al., 2013).

The barrier of illness or chronic disease may be viewed by some as nonmodifiable as well; however, the goal of medication or treatment adherence is to manage the illness or disease and gain quality of life. In the presence of dementia or cognitive function, this needs to be carefully assessed by the health care provider in order to understand the medical burden and capability of the client for self-management behaviors. The Mini-Mental State Examination (MMSE) can be administered by a health care provider to determine the cognitive function of the client

(Folstein, Folstein, & McHugh, 1975). In addition to cognitive function, depression plays a key role in medication adherence. The presence of symptoms or diagnosis of depression has been identified as an important correlation to low adherence to medication and treatment regimens (Holt et al., 2013). The presence of chronic diseases such as heart disease, chronic lung disease, hypertension, and diabetes, add more significant impacts to the client's everyday activities and lifestyle. The ongoing treatments, physician appointments, and self-care for these conditions can be a burden and decreases the client's motivation to process and understand complex medication regimens and treatment modalities. The health care provider should assess these barriers, along with health literacy, to gain a greater understanding of the client's current status. Identifying the underlying chronic disease and comorbid conditions allows the health care provider to assess barriers to medication adherence and have a greater understanding of how improved health literacy can assist the client to effectively manage chronic illness.

Tangible barriers to adherence are the obvious areas to focus on for the care of clients. These barriers include simple issues that are hopefully quick to avert, such as difficulty opening medication bottles and use of a pill box. However, there are larger issues such as polypharmacy and certainly health literacy is one area that health care providers and nurses can affect.

Polypharmacy is the use of multiple medications and/or the taking of more medications than are clinically needed (Lyles, Culver, Ivester, & Potter, 2013). This is a complication that contributes to poor health literacy in making the medication regimen more complex and difficult to understand. The prevalence of polypharmacy also contributes to a significant portion of health care expenditures. It is estimated by the Centers for Medicare and Medicaid Services that polypharmacy accounts for $50 billion annually in the United States (Lyles et al., 2013). Polypharmacy has also been linked to adverse drug reactions, functional impairments, and hospitalizations or even placements in nursing homes. As the largest cohort of medication consumers, older adults are at high risk for polypharmacy and complex medication and treatment regimens.

Poor health literacy is also one of the most significant barriers, and perhaps the most objective measure, that health care providers have the ability to affect. It is difficult to quantify the number or even percentage of older adults who have health literacy limitations. But consistently, research indicates that a majority of persons over the age of 65 years have some degree of health literacy limitation (Bauer et al., 2013; Lyles et al., 2013; Zamora & Clingerman, 2011). Consistently, the literature indicates that working to remove this modifiable barrier improves medication adherence (Grice et al., 2014; Lyles et al., 2013; O'Conor et al., 2015; Zhang et al., 2014). It is clear that improving a client's health literacy makes a difference; a difference that health care providers should pay attention to. For improving health care delivery and health outcomes for older adults, health literacy has become a national priority (Mosher, Lund, Kripalani, & Kaboli, 2012).

TECHNIQUES TO IMPROVE

With barriers identified, we can now focus on techniques to improve health literacy. Following a simplified version of many quality and nursing processes, improving health literacy can be approached in the process of **P**lanning, **I**mplementing, and **E**valuating. It's as easy as PIE! Well, maybe not quite that easy, but the mnemonic can help the health care provider guide the process of improving health literacy and serve as a reminder to keep it simple for the client.

P—Plan

Low health literacy can harm one's health, not only in understanding medications and managing chronic diseases, but also in the ability to fill out forms, participate in important screening tests, and take steps toward optimal health. This is especially true in older adults (National Library of Medicine, 2015) who may have lived with low health literacy for a long time and may need additional time or support to manage health care needs (Sorrell, 2006). When faced with a new diagnosis and treatment, or coping with the complexity of multiple illnesses, plan for additional time. As a health care provider, especially nurses, it feels as though not one more thing can fit into the day, so planning for additional time seems impossible. But keeping the "bigger picture" in mind for this population of clients is crucial. The additional time invested now could prevent an adverse effect of a medication, untoward health outcome or complication later. Addressing the adverse event later will most likely take more time, add more cost, and may cause greater harm to the older adult. Older adults are very capable, but they simply take more time. Their functional status does not allow them to move as fast and their cognitive function for new learning may be slower, but they are still able to learn new information and retain it (Cyr & Anderson, 2012). This becomes very important to older adults as they need their health status typically becomes more complex with age.

When assessing health literacy in older adult clients, two key elements the health care provider should remember are active listening and meeting them "right where they're at." Listening is important to the older adult group; they desire to be heard and not placed in a stereotypical image of a doddering old man or woman. It is essential that the health care provider ask questions about medications that are simple and clear. The health care provider should actively listen for ancillary information the client may also be providing in addition to answering a specific question. When providing instruction in taking medications and assessing if the medication is being taken correctly, the older adult may provide additional information that could assist in greater understanding of a potential health literacy issue. For example, the health care provider may ask about the five "rights" of medication administration—the right patient, right medication, right dose, right route (by mouth, topical, etc.), and the right time. If the client seems to hesitate when answering on the right dose and states that he or she has two different doses of the medication in the home, this is a gift of information! This allows the health care provider to ask if there are more than two different doses in the home, why (without placing judgement on the client), where they are kept in the home (same place or different), and if those different prescriptions are from different doctors.

Engaging with a client is another key element in working with older adults and adherence to medical regimens. "Meeting people where they're at" establishes a stronger health care provider–client relationship and thereby improves the overall health of the client (Woolhouse, Brown, & Thind, 2011). If a client isn't in a state of mind or being to learn new information about a medication, the health care provider can, and most likely will, overwhelm the client with too much, albeit stellar information. The older adult may be mentally preoccupied with a social situation in the family, a financial concern, a recent loss, or the health care provider's perception of him or her. The older adult may not have just a low health literacy level, but also a low educational level and cannot grasp more than one concept at a time. The health care provider that "tunes into" this situation and then breaks down the amount of information and states necessary information in the simplest of terms will have the greatest success in establishing a successful relationship with the client and achieving health goals. This requires that the plan, assessment, and ultimately the implementation toward medication adherence be highly individualized. While this takes additional time, practice will make it easier and more efficient. The care provider should develop a sophisticated and flexible approach to professional speaking and listening with clients.

As one ages, the complexity of health care needs tends to increase. Personalities become more diverse. There is more past life experience to influence the belief system. Taking time to learn who the client is becomes advantageous in the long term. This will help the health care provider to direct additional personnel to assist the client: the pharmacist for easy-open pill bottles or a service to fill a pill box or deliver medications to the home; the social worker to seek financial assistance for medications or provide counseling for a recent loss; or the medical equipment company for different options toward health care needs. Learning about the individual needs of the client assists in raising the health literacy of the older adult; the ultimate goal.

I—Implement

In completing your assessment of the older adult and planning how you will address health literacy needs and gain greater medication adherence, a principle of effectiveness comes to mind from Stephen Covey (1990) and The Seven Habits of Highly Effective People.

"Seek First to Understand, Then to Be Understood"

If you're like most people, you probably seek first to be understood; you want to get your point across. And in doing so, you may ignore the other person completely, pretend that you're listening, selectively hear only certain parts of the conversation or attentively focus on only the words being said, but miss the meaning entirely. So why does this happen? Because most people listen with the intent to reply, not to understand. You listen to yourself as you prepare in your mind what you are going to say, the questions you are going to ask, and so forth. You filter everything you hear through your life experiences, your frame of reference. You check what you hear against your autobiography and see how it measures up. And consequently, you decide prematurely what the other person means before he or she finishes communicating (Covey, 1990, p. 247).

As you implement your strategy for assessing health literacy, improving health literacy, and ultimately improving medication adherence, it is important to remember to work with smaller pieces of information. You can then increase the amount of information to work with as each individual is able to understand. As with any client, learning is unique to each individual. Speak in plain language that is easy for the older adult to understand (O'Conor et al., 2015). Although you as the health care provider have spent years learning a "medical language" or may have even taken a medical terminology class, the older adult most often has not. Additionally, there is most likely a generational gap with different terms for the same thing. It is an unreasonable expectation for the older adult to process and understand common abbreviations and terms used by nurses and physicians. Certainly learning them in one or two brief sessions is highly unreasonable. At the crossroads of medical jargon and health literacy, remember that this applies to prescriptions, appointments, instructions for tests, informed consents for procedures, calculations of doses involving mathematical ability or numeracy, and health teaching materials such as brochures and pamphlets. The individualization of these principles can be applied toward medical treatments and personal care for the benefit of the older adult as well.

In communicating with the client, there are some useful tools to assess readability levels and current health literacy levels. The SMOG readability formula is a common tool used to determine the readability level of health information that the health care provider is currently using or may develop as shown in Table 8.1 (Indian Health Service [IHS], 2015; McLaughlin, 1969).

This applies to written materials such as instruction sheets, pamphlets, brochures on medications, treatments, and/or procedures. The health care provider can perform this assessment quickly before giving information to an older adult client to see if this matches the level the client is able to understand. The health care provider could use this tool to identify if a brochure for a commonly used medication is appropriate for the older adult population. This is especially important to remember for more severe medications that if taken improperly, could have more serious adverse effects (MacLaughlin et al., 2005). The average reading level for all adults is about the eighth grade; however, for the vulnerable population of older adults, an estimated 40% read at the fifth grade level for literacy levels (U.S. Department of Health and Human Services, 2015). Health literacy then is a challenge for any reading materials above these grade levels. The SMOG formula is essential for anyone creating health education material for clients with perceived low health literacy. This allows the written material to be written at a low enough level that the large majority of older adults will be able to understand.

Another assessment tool to use with individuals to assess health literacy is the Rapid Estimate of Adult Literacy in Medicine-Short Form (REALM-SF). This is a shortened test of the original that has demonstrated reliability and validity as an efficient measure of health literacy skills, a prerequisite of self-care (Chin et al., 2011; Davis et al., 1993; Neilsen-Bohlman, Panzer, & Kindig, 2004). See Table 8.2.

TABLE 8.1 SMOG Readability Formula and Conversion Table (IHS, 2015)

Directions: Count 10 sentences in a row near the beginning of the material. Count 10 sentences in the middle. Count 10 sentences near the end (30 total sentences).

Count every word with three or more syllables in each group of sentences, even if the same word appears more than once.

Add the total number of words counted. Use the SMOG Conversion Table to find the grade level.

Word Counting Rules:
- A sentence is any group of words ending with a period, exclamation point, or question mark.
- Words with hyphens count as one word.
- Read numbers out loud to decide the number of syllables.
- Count abbreviations as the whole word they represent.

Word Count	Grade Level
0–2	4
3–6	5
7–12	6
13–20	7
21–30	8
31–42	9
43–56	10
57–72	11
73–90	12
91–110	13
111–132	14
133–156	15
157–182	16
183–210	17
211–240	18

TABLE 8.2 REALM-SF (AHRQ, 2015b)

Patient name _____ Date of birth_____ Reading level_____	
Date _____ Examiner _____ Grade completed _____	
Menopause	
Antibiotics	
Exercise	
Jaundice	
Rectal	
Anemia	
Behavior	

Instructions for Administering the REALM-SF:

1. Give the patient a copy of the REALM-SF form and score answers on a copy that is out of direct sight of the client. Hold the paper at an angle so that the patient is not distracted by your scoring.

2. Say: "I want to hear you read as many words as you can from this list. Begin with the first word and read aloud. When you come to a word you cannot read, do the best you can or say, 'blank' and go onto the next word."

3. If the patient takes more than 5 seconds on a word, say "blank" and point to the next word, if necessary, to move the patient along. If the patient begins to miss every word, have him or her pronounce only known words.

The use of the REALM assessment is very useful to the health provider before teaching a client in order to tailor to the individual need. In this brief screening instrument for health literacy, the client receives a point for every correct response according to the directions. This is a word recognition test, not a reading comprehension instrument. It is important to be strict and clear in administering and scoring the screening tool (AHRQ, 2015b). Make sure that the font size is appropriate for the client's visual capacity, a minimum of 18. Additionally, only count a word that is pronounced correctly in the form that it has been given. Certainly, the examiner has to allow for dialect and accents when working with clients who use English as a second language (AHRQ, 2015b). The test takes only about 2 to 3 minutes to administer and can provide valuable information in addressing health literacy. Using a tool such as REALM has proven to enhance health literacy and thereby improved overall health outcomes (Bauer et al., 2013; Chin et al., 2011).

E—Evaluate

In completing an evaluation of health literacy to gain greater understanding of health goals, it is helpful to get older adults to share in the goal of improved health literacy and optimal health outcomes. The outcomes of remaining in the community, having fewer adverse effects of medication (or none), or avoiding falls, for example, all need to be reinforced in moving forward in the process of ongoing assessment and evaluation of what is working and what is not. Return demonstration has been helpful, rather than relying on self-report in relation to processing the health education provided. This is a more objective measure in asking clients to show or demonstrate how they are completing a task rather than just reporting what they do.

Evaluation is a journey and not a destination. The health provider should be as objective as possible in assessing the client's understanding and processing of information without being obvious and perceived as "quizzing" the client, as this will not build trust in the health provider–client relationship. Throughout the process of evaluating, the provider should approach concepts in a collaborative manner that is individualized for the client. There are unique differences between a client that is an 86-year-old female who lives alone and is unsure of herself and a 70-year-old married, male veteran who is undaunted.

At every appointment, adherence should be checked, not necessarily by screening the client but making sure medications are being taken appropriately. This can be done by medication reconciliation either by a list of medications or a "brown bag" check. Medication reconciliation is completed by asking specific questions such as "When do you take this medication?" rather than "Are you taking your medications?" The health care provider should reconcile every medication on the health care provider's list to the list of medications the client possess. Any discrepancies should be addressed and corrected (Jones et al., 2014). The brown bag check is completed by the client actually bringing in the bottled medications in a "brown bag" and the health care provider performing a medication reconciliation, noting if the estimated appropriate number of pills are in the bottles indicating that the client has correctly taken the medication. This is not intended to check or spy on the older adult, but rather ensure that the current system established between the health care provider and client is effective. Phone calls to check on a client's progress in between appointments can be an effective tool of evaluation asking specific questions toward improved adherence and health literacy. As mentioned earlier, getting the client to a point of self-efficacy is a strong predictor of medication adherence in older adults (Chia et al., 2006).

IMPLICATIONS FOR NURSING

In the area of improving health literacy for older adults through adherence to medication and treatment regimens, nursing is a unique profession to address this issue effectively. Nurses care for older adults in many health care settings and are in an optimal position to improve health literacy across the continuum of care (Zamora & Clingerman, 2011). Caring for older adults requires a holistic approach due to the complexity of care that is needed and the diversity of each individual. Only nurses are educated in caring for clients in a holistic approach assessing each individual for that individual's response to illness (Scott-Tilley, Marshall-Gray, Valadez, & Green, 2005). Nurses are educated in a model of case management and coordinators of care interacting with multiple team members. Most frequently nurses have the most contact with the client, gaining the opportunity to establish a relationship with the client. A trusting relationship with the client allows for a more open and honest exchange of communication that may reveal a truer sense of health literacy skills possessed by the client. Although the techniques to assure adherence and raise health literacy can be done by all health care providers, nurses are key team members to complete REALM-SF screenings, perform medication reconciliation and, as advanced practice nurses, prescribe for and treat clients. As a professional nurse, assessment is consistently attached to the task. While some may see the nurse performing a task, the engaged nurse is also providing ongoing assessment of the client and the client's understanding of health care needs. Improving health care literacy demands this approach.

Professional nurses can also have a significant impact on shaping public policy in order to meet the health literacy needs of older adults (Zamora & Clingerman, 2011). Additional qualitative research is needed to understand the lived experiences of older adults as they navigate the management of chronic disease and complex medication and treatment regimes. As research may uncover more barriers to medication adherence or specific needs of subpopulations of older adults, nurses are best prepared to articulate the most innovative solutions to health literacy problems (Zamora & Clingerman, 2011).

CONCLUSIONS

There is evidence to support future trends and directions for enhanced medication adherence. Commonly used today are pill boxes and even phone services aligned with alert devices that will call clients and remind them to take medication. Newer developments in medication adherence techniques are telehealth devices and smartphone apps, both of which require additional costs to the client (Goldstein et al., 2014). This is not accessible to all clients. Most frequently, the lowest health literacy levels are found among lower socioeconomic groups and minority groups that may struggle with additional costs to enhance medication adherence. There is a need to strengthen the body of knowledge and evidence to see if these more costly methods actually improve medication adherence (Haugh, 2014). Improving health literacy for the older adults and removing barriers are less costly to the client and focus on the root issue of gaining greater understanding about medications and treatments.

As the older adult population continues to grow, the situation of medication adherence will not decrease, but only grow. It is estimated that by 2030, there will be over 70 million persons over the age of 65 years, more than ever before (Vincent & Velkoff, 2015). As a group they may experience more complexity in illness and more individualized therapy that will require higher levels of health literacy. The challenges for health care providers will continue to be many. Health care providers are vital to the evolving health literacy needs of this growing population.

The most commonly found definition of health literacy is "the degree to which individuals have the capacity to obtain, process, and understand basic health information and services needed to make appropriate health decisions" (Ratzan & Parker, 2015). However, Berkman, Davis, and Mcormack (2010) offer a slightly revised definition of health literacy to indicate perhaps a more accurate statement reflective of the overall goal: "Health literacy is the degree to which individuals can obtain, process, understand, and communicate about health-related information needed to make informed health decisions" (p. 16). Health literacy is the ability to get the health information one needs, and to understand it. It is also about using the information to make good decisions about optimal health and medical care.

REFERENCES

Agency for Healthcare Quality and Research. (2015a). *Advancing pharmacy health literacy practices through quality improvement*. Retrieved from http://www .ahrq.gov/professionals/education/curriculum-tools/pharmlitqi/resources.html

Agency for Healthcare Quality and Research. (2015b). *Rapid estimate of adult literacy in medicine-short form [REALM-SF]*. Retrieved from http://www.ahrq .gov/professionals/quality-patient-safety/quality-resources/tools/literacy/ realm.pdf

Bauer, A. M, Schillinger, D., Parker, M. M., Katon, W., Adler, N., Adams, A. S., . . . Karter, A. J. (2013). Health literacy and antidepressant medication adherence among adults with diabetes: The diabetes study of Northern California (DISTANCE). *Journal of General Internal Medicine*. 28(9): 1181–7. doi:10.1007/ s11606-013-2402-8

Berkman, N. D., Davis, T. C., & McCormack, L. (2010). Health literacy: What is it? *Journal of Health Communication, 15*(2), 9–19.

Chia, L., Schlenk, E. A., & Dunbar-Jacob, J. (2006). Effect of personal and cultural beliefs on medication adherence in the elderly. *Drugs Aging, 23*(3), 191–202.

Chin, J., Morrow, D. G., Stine-Morrow, E. A. L., Conner-Garcia, T., Graumlich, J. F., & Murray, M. D. (2011). The process-knowledge model of health literacy: Evidence from a componential analysis of two commonly used measures. *Journal of Health Communications, 16*, 222–241.

Covey, S. (1990). *The seven habits of highly effective people*. New York, NY: Free Press.

Cyr, A. A., & Anderson, N. D. (2012). Trial and error learning improves source learning among young and older adults. *Psychology of Aging, 27*(2), 429–439.

Davis, T. C., Long, S. W., Jackson, R. H., Mayeaux, E. J., George, R. B., Murphy, P. W., & Crouch, M. A. (1993). Rapid estimate of adult literacy in medicine: A shortened screening instrument. *Family Medicine, 25*, 391–395.

Folstein, M. F., Folstein, S. E., & McHugh, P. R. (1975). Mini-mental state: A practical method of grading the state of patients for the clinician. *Journal of Psychiatric Research, 12*, 1081–1091.

Goldstein, C. M., Gathright, E. C., Dolansky, A., Gunstad, J., Sterns, A., Redle, J. D., . . . Hughes, J. N. (2014). Randomized controlled feasibility trial of two telemedicine reminder systems for older adults with heart failure. *Journal of Telemedicine and Telecare, 20*(6), 293–299.

Grice, G. R., Tiemeier, A., Hurd, P., Berry, T., Voorhees, M., Prosser, T. R, . . . Duncan, W. (2014). Student use of health literacy tools to improve patient understanding and medication adherence. *Consultant Pharmacist, 29*(4), 240–253.

Haugh, K. H. (2014). Medication adherence in older adults: The pillbox half full. *Nurse Clinics of North America, 49*, 183–199.

Holt, E., Joyce, C., Dornelles, A., Morisky, D., Webber, L. S., Muntner, P., & Krousel-Wood, M. (2013). Sex differences in barriers to antihypertensive medication adherence: Findings from the cohort study of medication adherence among older adults. *Journal of the American Geriatrics Society, 61*(4), 558–564.

Indian Health Service. (2015). Patient-provider communication toolkit. Retrieved from https://www.ihs.gov/healthcommunications/documents/toolkit/Tool13.pdf

Jones, J. H., Treiber, L. A., & Jones, M. C. (2014). Intervening at the intersection of medication adherence and health literacy. *Journal for Nurse Practitioners, 10*(8), 527–534.

Loke, Y. K., Hinz, I., Wang, X., & Salter, C. (2012). Systematic review of consistency between adherence to cardiovascular or diabetes medication and health literacy in older adults. *Annals of Pharmacotherapy, 6*(46), 863–872.

Lyles, A., Culver, N., Ivester, J., & Potter, T. (2013). Effects of health literacy and polypharmacy on medication adherence. *Consultant Pharmacist, 28*(12), 793–799.

MacLaughlin, E. J., Raehl, C. L., Treadway, A. K., Sterling, T. L., Zoller, D. P., & Bond, C. A. (2015). Assessing medication adherence in the elderly: Which tools to use in clinical practice. *Drugs Aging, 22*(3), 231–255.

McLaughlin, G. H. (1969). SMOG grading: A new reading formula. *Journal of Reading, 12*, 639–640.

Mosher, H. J., Lund, B. C., Kripalani, S., & Kaboli, P. J. (2012). Association of health literacy with medication knowledge, adherence, and adverse drug events among elderly veterans. *Journal of Health Communications, 17*, 241–251.

National Council on Aging. (2015). *Chronic disease.* Retrieved from https://www.ncoa.org/healthy-aging/chronic-disease

National Library of Medicine. (2015). *Health literacy.* Retrieved from https://vsearch.nlm.nih.gov/vivisimo/cgi-bin/query-meta?query=health+literacy&v%3Aproject=nlm-main-website

Neilsen-Bohlman, L., Panzer, A. M., & Kindig, D. A. (2004). *Health literacy: A prescription to end confusion* (Institute of Medicine Report). Washington, DC: National Academies Press.

O'Conor, R., Wolf, M. S., Smith, S. G., Martynenko, M., Vecencio, D. P., Sano, M., . . . Federman, A. D. (2015). Health literacy, cognitive function, proper use, and adherence to inhaled asthma controller medications among older adults with asthma. *Chest, 147*(5), 1307–1315.

Ratzan, S., & Parker, R. (2015). *Health literacy and older adults.* United States Department of Health and Human Services. Retrieved from http://www.health.gov/communication/literacy/olderadults/literacy.htm#p3

Scott-Tilley, D., Marshall-Gray, P., Valadez, A., & Green, A. (2005). Integrating long-term care concepts into baccalaureate nursing education: The road to quality geriatric health care. *Journal of Nursing Education, 44*(6), 286–290.

Sirey, J. A., Bruce, M. L., & Alexopoulos, G. S. (2001). Stigma as a barrier to recovery: Perceived stigma and patient-rated severity of illness as predictors of antidepressant drug adherence. *Psychiatric Services, 52*, 1615–1620.

Sirey, J. A., Greenfield, A., Weinberger, M. K., & Bruce, M. L. (2013). Medication beliefs and self-reported adherence among community-dwelling older adults. *Clinical Therapeutics, 35*(2), 153–160.

Sorrell, J. M. (2006). Health literacy in older adults. *Journal of Psychosocial Nursing, 44*(3), 17–20.

U.S. Department of Health and Human Services. (2015). Health resources and services administration: Health literacy. Retrieved from http://www.hrsa.gov/publichealth/healthliteracy/index.html

Vincent, G. K., & Velkoff, V. A. (2015). *The next four decades: The older population in the United States 2010–2050.* Retrieved from http://www.census.gov/prod/2010pubs/p25–1138.pdf

Woolhouse, S., Brown, J. B., & Thind, A. (2011). 'Meeting people where they're at': Experiences of family physicians engaging women who use illicit drugs. *Annals of Family Medicine, 9*(3), 244–249.

Zamora, H., & Clingerman, E. M. (2011). Health literacy among older adults: A systematic literature review. *Gerontological Nursing, 37*(10), 41–51.

Zhang, N. J., Terry, A., & McHorney, C. A. (2014). Impact of health literacy on medication adherence: A systematic review and meta-analysis. *Annals of Pharmacotherapy, 48*(6), 741–751.

CHAPTER 9

Health Literacy and Speech and Hearing Professionals

CATHLEEN CARNEY-THOMAS

Health literacy is limited not only to a person's ability to read but how well a person can understand, comprehend, and remember the spoken word. If a person presents with a communication disorder, it can make the task of understanding and recalling health information even more difficult. It is widely shown that being able to understand health information and make appropriate decisions are paramount to a person's well-being. Functional health literacy skills are instrumental to participation in patient-centered care. It is often the speech language pathologists and audiologists who are at the forefront assessing and treating people who present to our doctors' offices, nursing homes, hospitals, and rehabilitation centers with speech and hearing impairments and often reduced health literacy abilities. Most current research into communication risk or education about health decisions has not included people with disabilities.

SPEECH AND HEARING PROFESSIONALS AS HEALTH LITERACY ADVOCATES

Speech language pathologists and audiologists hold certification in the speech and hearing field through the American Speech Language Hearing Association [ASHA]. Considered the specialists in human communication, speech pathologists and audiologists can add expertize to the skills of communicating complex medical messages to the individuals who present with limited health literacy skills. And as part of the organization and health care team, these speech and hearing professionals work to insure that consumer messages incorporate health literacy principles so that the work of speech pathologists and audiologists can be understood by and utilized by the widest audience possible. ASHA's vision statement includes principles for "making effective communication a human right accessible and achievable by all" (American Speech Language Hearing Association [ASHA], 2008).

People with communication disabilities include individuals who have impairments in-body functions of hearing, vision, speech, language, and cognition and body structures of facial expression, body language, gesture, sign, and Braille. Impairments are also influenced by the degree of the impairment, whether mild or severe, and the communication activity of listening, speaking, reading, writing, or gesturing. People will fall into four distinct categories: those with a pre-existing disability of communication, for example, Down's syndrome, cerebral palsy, and autism; those with a secondary sudden onset of symptoms—some diagnoses include cerebral vascular accident (stroke) and traumatic brain injury; those with a communication disability secondary to a medical intervention; and those who have experienced laryngeal surgery, tracheostomy, or medication delirium (Ottalloran, Hickson, & Worrall, 2007). There is also a group of individuals who present with a reduction in communication skills due to the gradual deterioration of cognitive skills, those individuals diagnosed with mild cognitive impairment, and Alzheimer's dementia.

People with communication disorders are at risk of not being able to communicate in the health care environment effectively. Not only are they vulnerable due to the illness but they are also trying to communicate in an unfamiliar environment. The consequence is receipt of suboptimal care and poorer long-term health outcomes than those without communication disorders. In terms of individual factors, it is known that individuals with speech, language, visual, hearing, and intellectual disabilities experience even greater challenges when they need to apply literacy skills (Wuhlisch & Pascoe, 2011).

According to current information, one in six Americans has a communication disorder. The elderly are often diagnosed with communication disorders due to diseases common with aging or due to preexisting conditions exacerbated by typical aging. Communication disorders include deafness, people with hearing loss, language delay, developmental disorders, autism spectrum disorders, aphasia, stuttering, auditory perception and processing disorders, mild cognitive impairments, and traumatic brain injury. These individuals present to the speech and hearing professional with unique challenges to tailor the message to the specific strategies that are individualized to the specific strengths and needs of the clients. The link between communication impairments typical with these disorders and health literacy skills is frequently not considered. Often health literacy and communication deficits will be over- or under-recognized by other health providers and contribute to the inability of our clients to gather adequate health information and fully participate in treatment regimens (Allen, 2005; ASHA, 2008).

To the speech language pathologist, literacy in the primary mode is face-to-face or spoken language. The secondary mode is the representation of print or written language. All language is viewed within a context. Communication exchanges are considered natural and redundant. In spoken language there is the use of overlapping cues, both verbal and nonverbal, used to minimize misunderstandings. In spoken language, if a breakdown occurs, the speaker is able to repeat the sentence, gesture, pantomime, rephrase, use concrete examples, demonstrate, or explain with visual supports. Spoken language is contextualized and is grounded in the here and now. It is concrete; the speaker and the listener will share the same knowledge, background, or experience. Once language becomes written, it becomes decontextualized. Breakdowns in comprehension go unnoticed and misunderstandings cannot be immediately repaired. Reading comprehension varies with the individual familiarity of the *context* of the text. Again, language is viewed within the context or the experience of the language message.

Disciplines in health care rely on health literacy that includes all types of communication, theory, practice, health education, cultural competency, public health, organizational, and systems analysis. The tasks involved in the practice of speech pathology and audiology also include assessments of receptive skills for oral language including tasks for auditory comprehension, such as answering yes/no questions, processing, and following verbally presented directions. Clinical decisions are made with the data and scores to assess reading skills at word, phrase, and sentence levels, and whether to do oral or silent reading. Expressive skills for the production of oral language include the tasks of naming pictures, performing cloze tasks, and answering "wh" questions. Again, dependent on receptive and expressive language and reading skills, written expression may or may not be assessed. Cognitive skills are also considered. Assessments of sustained attention, memory, problem solving, and reasoning are provided. It should be noted that deficits in oral literacy (receptive and expressive language) or language within a context are firm indicators of deficits at least equal to or more depressed in written literacy or decontextualized language.

Assessment data provides the speech and language professional with baseline abilities of communication skills for the client that are used to determine the strategies to be targeted to strengthen functional communication skills. Baseline communication scores also provide the speech and hearing professional with supporting information for the type of learning style and the best methods for teaching functional tasks for use once discharged from therapy. These tasks may also include treatment strategies for increasing word understanding, direction following, word recall, answering questions, and deciphering the meaning of signs, sounds, and symbols.

Speech and hearing professionals also have to be involved in relaying messages for the clients to give informed consent for the treatment plan set forth, and be involved in giving and taking case histories of communication-impaired clients. Knowing the prior level of functioning, educational background, employment skills, hobbies, and activities of daily living allow health care professionals to place more emphasis on the communication context or experience of the client. Speech language pathologists are required to request information prior to initiation of assessment or treatments. Frequently due to HIPPA, laws make it difficult to request this information from significant others. The use of picture-based communication tools during preadmission screening could provide the multidisciplinary team with basic information to guide these initial conversations.

Patient information leaflets play an important role in the provision of speech and language therapy. There is widespread use of written information to help with supporting information regarding the topics discussed in treatment as well as the lifestyle decisions and changes that may have to take place as part of the rehabilitation process. Yet, these leaflets are of variable quality. Written information is an important tool in the health care rehabilitative process; however, when providing them to the client, the professional must be aware of the patient's abilities to read, comprehend, analyze, decode instructions, recognize symbols, charts, diagrams, and the ability to understand risks and benefits of treatments offered to them (Allen, 2005; Pothier, Day, Harris, & Pothier, 2008). Literacy and language goes beyond simple patient–doctor interactions. Health professionals should make it a priority to gather suggestions from the speech, hearing, and communication specialists to better understand clients' skills in health literacy.

Speech and hearing professionals have a reciprocal responsibility in health literacy. As mentioned previously in this chapter, speech and hearing professionals screen for, test, and evaluate the severity of communication/health literacy skills. They also provide treatment to improve these communication/language/literacy deficits. Many believe it is possible to "fix" the communication deficit of the individual. Improvements can be made with treatments; however, it is likely that the incidence of poor health literacy skills persists or increases as a person ages regardless of any medical condition. Age-related changes in visual and cognitive skills impact the reading skills. In reality, strategies and techniques employed or used by Speech Hearing professionals do not always take into account matching the expectations and preferences to the skill set of the elderly client providing the information. Speech and language treatment refers to the therapy that aims to bring about a positive change in the client's communication skills. Speech pathologists frequently provide large amounts of information to clients with the assumption that they already have the reasoning for the importance of the intervention and the need for change. The buy into the therapy approach means that the client is able to act upon the strategies needed for change. This involves all aspects of the language continuum with hearing, processing, understanding, responding, critically thinking, and applying the context to create experiences (Griffin, Mc Kenna, & Tooth, 2003; Wuhlisch & Pascoe, 2011).

In speech and hearing as well as other health care professions, client education is the most commonly used treatment medium. It is used as both a treatment strategy and as a way to enhance and share the treatment process. Speech and hearing professionals often work to teach clients skills and techniques to deal with and adjust to life with a particular condition, do exercises, manage stress, and use adaptive equipment. Speech language pathologists provide written information to the client as a means to facilitation of the collaborative approach to care (McKenna & Scott, 2007).

Client recall of oral information is often inadequate, with clients recalling only 35% of information provided orally. Written information then becomes the most common material added to the oral teaching as it offers message *consistency* (Griffin, et al., 2003). Of course one of the aims used in therapy is to provide the client with comprehensive information about a topic, but the importance of the readability of the text provided may be overlooked. Readability is a measurement of literacy as it goes up (gets harder) the comprehension is reduced. Consistency of the information adds to reinforcement or adding to the context of messages (Pothier et al., 2008).

SPEECH AND HEARING PROFESSIONALS: SCOPE OF PRACTICE IN HEALTH LITERACY

As the specialists who assess for communication disorders and disabilities, there are formalized, standardized assessments that are performed and relayed as definitive measures of each client's language skills. Oral language skill is of critical concern because public health communication relies on oral communication to convey health information to the public. Written language skills, or health literacy is of concern for follow-up, generalization, and offers several advantages to the client.

The limitations of commonly used health literacy assessments as well as some standardized speech and language assessments are similar. The Test of Functional Health Literacy in Adults [TOFHLA] requires a performance through 100 items for reading comprehension and numeracy related to medical instruction and prescription labels. The length of the test is of concern due to the inability of many to attend for longer times, as well as the difficulty of reading level due to unfamiliarity of the terminology used. The information is not tested within the context and renders the grade level markers unreliable. The Rapid Estimate of Adult Literacy in Medicine [REALM] requires performing a word recognition test of 26 words and requires the client to orally read each word. The speech language pathologist will test for both oral and silent reading abilities as silent reading is easier than oral reading and the two skill levels may not be used as an equal measure of function of health literacy (McCrary & Hester, 2011). These health literacy assessments are often limited to print literacy and do not take into account the listening and speaking skills of the patient (Hester & Ratchford, 2009). Several other limitations have been noted, aside from the length of the test, from the complexity of the reading level to the assessment of only single words and not sentences. Current health literacy assessments do not assess the entire spectrum of health literacy that includes speaking and listening. The results of a comprehensive speech and language evaluation should be included in all records for our elderly to augment the information health care professionals have regarding the clients' functional skills.

However, health literacy involves other skills such as cultural and conceptual knowledge and listening and speaking. The focus on only health terms has been criticized as well, in that many of the other materials that must be read do not involve use of medical terms. Language usage or word usage is based on each person's lexicon or store of words held in memory. Word order determines the meaning of the word that should be accepted. Dynamic measures of the client's language skills should be done at regular intervals as the level may change over time. Even for clients with adequate health literacy and language skills, written information should never replace oral information (Griffin et al., 2003; Hester & Ratchford, 2009).

Speech and hearing professionals often look to language and communication areas that affect literacy and attempt to use them to affect changes in the methods of viewing and accommodating health literacy–challenged clients. One such model is the pragmatic model which emphasizes the social use of language.

The pragmatic model applies to the study of variations in the communication intentions of patient–provider interactions. Consideration of the client's ability to study and ask questions as investigation of the types of questioning and communication intentions may add more information about the health literacy of the client and therefore expected health outcomes. Investigations of the questioning and communicative intentions may also reveal information regarding the client's communication skills within the health care system (Hester & Ratchford, 2009).

There is also the cognitive science model that includes the syntax (word order or grammar) and semantics (word use or lexicon) of the health communications. In viewing the syntactic complexity of both the written and spoken statements, the readability and understandability can be noted and possibly changed for better patient understanding. Passive conversational type statements are more readily understood. The syntactic complexity of the statements provided are a challenge as well to the clients who present with communication deficits and lower health literacy. Also part of the cognitive model is the problem-solving use with the level of abstract language given. The client's ability to make complex inferences with this speech and health literacy information is dependent on understanding the way in which the language is used or the meaning behind the words. The context based on the client's experiences comes into play. The combination in use of the cognitive and social model skills leads to motivation and ability of the individual to act upon, or understand and use the information effectively, which leads to empowerment (Hester & Ratchford, 2009).

Health providers commonly use written material as a low-cost approach to providing patients with health information, but rehabilitation professionals are rarely trained in the skills of preparing written health information using the principles of health literacy, or in evaluating such materials. Yet part of the best practices of rehabilitation professionals includes provision of home programs and exercise regimens for the client to maintain. Education beyond the therapy session has been shown to improve client satisfaction, knowledge, adherence to treatment, physiological outcomes, and increased self-management. The principles of adult education show that visual and auditory modes of communication may be the most effective in conveying the information because they encompass different learning styles. Best practices state that the information should be patient oriented and designed for individual needs. These health information materials can be effective only if they can be read, understood, and remembered by the patient (Hoffman & Wordall, 2004).

Providers cannot assume that the information they receive from the professional organization or government is acceptable for all. The U.S. health system operates largely on the assumption that all patients have high English language literacy skills. All health care providers must ask the questions: Is the information right for the patient; Is the message consistent with what you want to relay; and Is the information complete? (Hasselkus, 2009; Rao, 2007).

KNOWLEDGE OF PATIENTS' HEALTH LITERACY

Health professionals tend to have little awareness of clients' reading difficulties because of their own level of education and because they assume they will be able to recognize those who present with poor literacy skills. This is often not the case due to the strategies clients with poor literacy skills use to conceal their reading disabilities. Direct questioning of reading abilities can be done (Griffin et al., 2003); however, even physicians tend to incorrectly classify reading skills and/or patients denying they a reading difficulty.

Most people with limited literary skills compensate in other ways. The most common is inviting family members to accompany them to the doctor's office. They also feel a strong stigma attached to limited reading and writing skills and conceal the fact they cannot read—often stating something simple such as: "I forgot my glasses"; "My handwriting is not good"; or "I forgot to bring my information with me. Can I take it home?" (U.S. Department of Health and Human Services [USDHHS], 2014). The knowledge and skills of the health care provider are an important concern as there must be the awareness of the need for nontechnical assistance. The provider should note those patients who need assistance or privacy filling out forms, and guidance getting to and from the waiting room, where food and drink are being placed. Staff must also be aware of how to use alternative augmentative communication devices (Ottalloran et al., 2007).

When working with the elderly population, common disorders or symptoms seen are related to changes in brain function from disease or atrophy. Two prevalent disorders that speech and hearing professionals treat are aphasia and cognitive decline from dementia.

APHASIA

Aphasia is an acquired neurogenic impairment of language resulting from focal brain damage in the left hemisphere or language area of the brain. Cerebral vascular accident, often referred to as a "stroke," is the most common cause. The diagnosis of aphasia does not include the motor disorders that also may co-occur. Communication deficits can be present in all areas of input: hearing, understanding, and reading as well as the output modalities: speaking and writing (Doyle et al., 2013). Part of the speech and hearing professional's scope of practice is to educate the client on the lifestyle changes that may need to occur during the recovery process; the stroke information leaflets provided are often at reading levels above that of the stroke survivor's level (Pothier et al., 2008).

Older people with aphasia tend to participate in the same types of communication activities as healthy older people but differences are noted in the frequency of these activities and the fewer number of communication partners. Fewer partners limit the pragmatic or social aspect of the language learning, making placing within a context more difficult. Those with aphasia had fewer instances of story-telling, writing, suggesting, acknowledging, questioning, bargaining, joking, commenting, or sharing their life stories. For those with aphasia, the conversation tended to focus on the here and now and relate to people in their restricted social networks (Davidson, Worall, & Hickson, 2003). Reading materials for people with aphasia tend to be newspapers, TV guides, mail, bank statements, and pamphlets. Significant others tend to notice some communication breakdowns during these tasks and often use gestures or pantomime strategies, not verbal language, to help comprehension.

One aspect of the inpatient protocol with a person with aphasia is to determine if the patient understands his or her regimen for medication prior to discharge. The patient should be able to count out pills, identify when they are to be taken, and understand any other requirements for the routine. Patient rights should be taught as well. Speech and hearing clinicians should participate in all staff training as well as evaluate the signage in the facility. All staff should be alert to cues of misspellings and incomplete forms. The speech language pathologist can integrate safety and enhanced literacy and improved compliance as part of the treatment program and encourage the family members and the patients to ask questions and be sure that they understand. Each session's closing questions to the patient should be: "Do you have any questions?" (Rao, 2007). Diaries can be used to monitor skills in reading and writing. Diaries or daily journals help integrate the health education changes into the client's regular routine or help provide a context to the information. Diaries should be reviewed in an oral or conversational context.

The measurement systems that are used to determine readability often rely too much on a client's language skills. The cloze procedure, for example, deletes words from text and asks readers to fill in the blanks. When the percentage of correct insertions is calculated, it does come closer to determining true understanding of the text, but its results are dependent on the client's premorbid language skills. Often, pictures are used to impact the readability and the understandability of the words; however, a recent study found that pictures do not necessarily improve understanding in readers with aphasia, especially if clip art was used (Pothier et al., 2008). Clients who present with aphasia will respond to the use of the actual item or object over the use of a picture. The client can then discover the function or use during role play, gesture, or pantomime, based on previous experiences with it.

COGNITIVE DEFICITS—DEMENTIA

Dementia is considered a disease process resulting in cognitive loss versus a disability with a person able to provide some information regarding his or her own quality of life (Ottalloran, et al., 2007). Older adults with cognitive brain impairment have difficulty with short-term memory. One memory strategy often taught is to reduce the number of words that can be processed and placed into short-term memory, which will aide the client in picking out the salient concepts or words that need to be recalled. Review and repetition improves the ability to move information from short-term memory into working memory, and this can be accomplished by adding a conclusion and a summary at the end of a paragraph (Griffin et al., 2003). Cognitive limitations often contribute to language impairments and the ability to "code switch." Code switching is part of the pragmatic model of communication and requires the client to understand the sender's experience or context. Clients with dementia are unable to take the other's experience as their own.

Older people 65 years and over have the lowest level of functional literacy when compared to any other age group. Literacy skills markedly decline with age as reading encompasses several visual and cognitive abilities—acuity and tracking as well as abilities to attend and concentrate, recognize and remember words and phrases, and execute information-processing skills. It is possible that reading is affected by even mild cognitive decline. Elders tend to read less informative documents and health literacy follows the "use it or lose it" assumption. Deficiencies seen are the omitted relevant information, failure to give balanced a view of treatment options, and avoidance of discussing uncertainties (Griffin et al., 2003).

Communication skills and social networks change with age. Speech and hearing professionals should investigate the changes in language with the older population to determine if the changes are functionally or clinically relevant. Do these changes make a difference in the quality of life of our elders or do they need to be adjusted with age? With this population, we use mostly low-tech strategies and view poor outcomes as being related to the clients themselves and compliance. It is doubtful that one can represent language information internally without exposure to the experience.

CURRENT CONCERNS

Difficulties with health literacy of the patients can add to the risk management issues of speech and hearing professionals as well as the administration of the facility. Those with limited health literacy have delayed disgnoses or difficulty using preventative health services. Those with limited health literacy have difficulty in navigating the health care system, which leads to no-shows, insurance eligibility problems, and incomplete or inaccurate forms. There are the therapeutic failures from incomplete or inaccurate medical records leading to incorrect diagnoses and an increased malpractice risk (Rao, 2007). Dealing with health literacy is a legal necessity as it empowers the clients, helps them assume responsibility, and increases client and family satisfaction.

Often our clients have to recall information from other professionals first—for example, the ENT physician for voice consults and referral after the laryngectomy. The information is too complex and they are overwhelmed. Some clients may come in only once a month, or very infrequently, for follow up. They have difficulty attending appointments; they have a fear of failing; they hamper the flow of feedback and feel helpless; and are often scared to tell the clinician they don't understand. Information often gets lost between caregivers, leading to difficulty with follow-up after discharge (Wuhlisch & Pascoe, 2011).

CURRENT INTERVENTIONS

The most immediately used response is the Universal Precautions Approach—meaning we should teach all clients in the same simple language manner regardless of health literacy level. We should request that clients review information with a significant other prior to making discharge decisions (Critilli & Schaefer, 2011). People can take in only so much information before the short-term memory is overloaded.

To date, interventions found useful for helping those with limited health literacy achieve better patient outcomes and safety are the teach-back technique, multimedia supports, simple language, support persons and experiences, and assisted or choral reading. Put "tell me" in front of the questions or add prompts (Critilli & Schaefer, 2011). Communication specialists can add to the concept of empowerment by teaching patients and clients about the skills that facilitate health communications (Hester & Ratchford, 2009).

FUTURE DIRECTIONS

Speech language pathologists should begin researching and testing subjective measures of health information understanding for all clients. Using the concepts of language in conversational context, speech and hearing professionals can develop screening questions for a small number of sensitive questions that could identify patients at risk for reduced health literacy. Training for all staff should be provided on a regular basis. Staff can develop skills in observation of specific behaviors that could show limits of health literacy for each client. Providing methods for staff notations in charting and health records that would specify communication limitations, so other health care providers could modify their interactions, would aid in the ability of clients to read, understand, and use the health information provided. During case history and admission assessment, having a list of specific questions geared toward the continuum of health literacy for oral and written language skills, would help identify those able to provide adequate background information.

The background information can be used to help health care providers understand the client's overall communication level as well as the client's abilities for health reasoning and problem solving and ability to advocate (Hester & Ratchford, 2009; Wuhlisch & Pascoe, 2011).

Frequently, clinicians have been taught to use the teach-back approach; however, this often has time constraints. The client may forget key pieces of information. So the clinician must frequently ask: "Do you understand?" This type of closed-ended question often elicits positive answers whether the client understands or not. Health information provided in written as well as verbal forms will add to the client's ability to use several learning styles. When the health care professional uses auditory and visual techniques at the same time, it is more likely the client will understand and process the information provided. The teach-back method must be done within *context* maintaining an interactive communication loop. Speech and hearing professionals are trained to use everyday functional examples to aid communication skills. For the client who is communication impaired, the ability to restate in his or her own words may be lost. Many may simply repeat what is heard without comprehension of the concepts; however, having the client act out or demonstrate understanding may prove a more accurate approach to determining understanding and follow through. For clients with a higher level of verbal communication skills, using the teach-back strategy and the strategy of "Ask Me 3" may be an additional alternative, as it prompts patients to ask their providers three questions: What is my main problem? What do I need to do? Why is it important for me to do this? These techniques can also be used in training the caregivers and significant others to aid in follow through and compliance with home exercise programs (Critilli & Schaefer, 2011; USDHHS, 2014).

The common practice to educate verbally should be reinforced with written materials. Written materials have an advantage of being able to refresh the person's memory as needed, along with memory strategies provided as part of the speech and language interventions. Clients appreciate written materials as well. Questions and requests of clarification usually come after the client has visited the health care professional, not during the visit. Written material within a context of experience can guide the client and caregiver to the amount and level of information as the coping skills increase (Hoffman & Wordall, 2004).

Many health care professionals have the need to provide health information to their aging clients. Using the language and literacy skill knowledge of the speech and hearing professional in the development and dissemination of health information regarding dysphagia, hearing loss, laryngectomy, tracheostomy, traumatic brain injury, and aphasia would increase readability and understanding of the information. Speech language pathologists should consider designing the materials themselves. As rehabilitation professionals, they must become critical consumers of the material and review and appraise for quality and effectiveness (Griffin et al., 2003). Written materials should discuss the what, why, and when. A reciprocal/conversational approach is necessary to help encourage decision making. Use of conversational tone during this review of materials should also include checklists and open ended questions to increase the understanding of the information.

Interdisciplinary and transdisciplinary teams should provide advice and guidance to the development of health literacy curricula in the university for speech language pathologists and audiologists as it pertains to services provided (McCrary & Hester, 2011). Coursework, such as that provided in this text, should be part of every student's and future professional's curriculum when working with the elderly client.

Speech and hearing professionals have been taught "the six steps" in guiding clients to a better understanding of health information. (1) Slow down and consider a patient-centered approach. Often clients presenting with chronic communication disorders need additional time to process and retrieve the verbal information needed to respond. Possibly the use of cues and prompts aid the ability of the client to process and use the information provided. (2) Use plain, nonmedical language without medical jargon. Chronic communication disorders inhibit the ability to learn new complex words easily, so these clients rely on the word store or lexicon developed through personal experience. Naming pictures or describing item is not functional learning for our elderly as it is not able to be put into the context of personal experience. (3) Request demonstrating and/or drawing pictures. Those who are nonverbal or difficult to understand due to oral muscle weakness may be able to provide pictorial information on paper without the added stress of using words. (4) Limit the amount of information and repeat it, using the "Teach-Back" or "Show Me Method." (5) Design short and long-term communication goals to use the information from the patient educational material within the clinical setting. And, lastly, create a shame-free environment (Rao, 2007). Allowing the client to feel successful in the treatment session, providing strategies to help the communication process, and recalling the information (generalizing) from other areas keeps the conversation and the context of the communication active throughout the therapeutic process.

Issues around client health literacy and recall of information and how these can be overcome should be viewed in the area of developing context. Speech language therapy refers to the treatment that aims to bring about positive change in the communication of individuals. Utilization of the pragmatic approach (social conversational approach in a context) as well as the cognitive approach (semantics, syntax, and problem solving) has been shown to be the most beneficial for those with declining health literacy skills. Health care professionals should consider providing the information over time. Breaking the information down into immediately relevant steps that can be applied gradually to the lifestyle changes is one of the strategies employed by speech language pathologists to help in memory, carry over, and buy in. The speech and hearing professional can act as mediator to interpret available data and information and present back to the client with appropriate strategies for comprehension and recall so functional lifestyle change can be brought about (Wuhlisch & Pascoe, 2011).

Developing literacy skills within a context assumes that the flow of information has no starting or stopping point. The information becomes useful in the daily routine, adding to the elder client's experience and therefore making the context of the communication relevant whether in oral or written form.

REFERENCES

Allen, M. (2005). What is health literacy? *Access Audiology, 4*(1). Retrieved from www.asha.org/aud/articles/healthlit/

American Speech Language Hearing Association (ASHA). (2008). *Clinical supervision in speech language pathology (position statement)*. Retrieved from www.asha.org/policy

Critilli, C., & Schaefer, C. (2011, July/August). Case studies in geriatric health literacy. *Orthopaedic Nursing, 30*(4), 281–285.

Davidson, B., Worall, L., & Hickson, L. (2003). Identifying the communication activities of older people with aphasia: Evidence for naturalistic observations. *Aphasiology, 17*(3), 243–264.

Doyle, P., Hula, W., Hula-Amsterdam, S., Stone, C., Wormbaugh, J., Ross, K., & Shumaker, J. (2013). Self and surrogate reported communication functioning in Aphasia. *Quality Life Resources, 22*, 957–967.

Griffin, J., McKenna, K., & Tooth, L. (2003). Written health education materials: Making them more effective. *Australian Occupational Therapy Journal, 50*, 170–177.

Hasselkus, A. (2009, June 20). Health literacy in clinical practice. *The ASHA Leader, 14*, 28–29.

Hester, E., & Ratchford, R. (2009). Health literacy and the role of the SLP. *American Journal of Speech Language Pathology, 18*, 180–193.

Hoffman, T., & Wordall, L. (2004). Designing effective written health educational materials: Considerations for health professionals. *Disabilities and Rehabilitation, 26*(19), 1166–1173.

McCrary, M., & Hester, E. (2011). Health literacy and multicultural populations. *Perspectives for Communication Disorders and Services in Culturally and Linguistically Diverse Populations, 18,* 79–87.

McKenna, K., & Scott, J. (2007). Do written materials that use content design principles improve older people's knowledge? *Australian Occupational Therapy Journal, 54,* 102–113.

Ottalloran, R., Hickson, L., & Worrall, L. (2007). Environmental factors that influence communication between people with communication disability and their healthcare providers in hospital: A review of the literature within the International Class of Function Disability and Health (ICF) framework. *International Journal of Language and Communication Disorders, 43*(6), 601–632.

Pothier, L., Day, R., Harris, C., & Pothier, D. (2008). Readability statistics of patient information leaflets in a speech and language therapy department. *International Journal Language Communication Disorders, 43*(6), 712–722.

Rao, P. (2007, May 8). Health literacy: The cornerstone of patient safety. *The ASHA Leader, 12,* 8–12.

U.S. Department of Health and Human Services (USDHHS). (2014). *About health literacy.* Retrieved from www.health.gov/communication/literacy

Wuhlisch, F., & Pascoe, M. (2011). Maximizing health literacy and client recall in developing context: Speech language therapists and client perspective. *International Journal Language and Communication Disorders, 46*(5), 592–607.

CHAPTER 10

Improving Health Literacy and Health Outcomes Using Cognitive Prosthetic Devices

ANTHONY A. STERNS AND TRACY A. RILEY

Quantum advances in health-related discoveries have dramatically affected the process of providing health care. For example, once terminal conditions have become lifelong chronic conditions such as with HIV infection. Complicated treatment regimens have been simplified in order to increase efficacy and adherence to those treatments. The health care system itself has experienced significant change including the recent focus on primary or preventive health initiatives outside the clinical setting.

While advances in science have been made, there has been insufficient recognition of the importance of health literacy for recipients of health care. There are at least two requisite conditions when using patient-centered approaches for any health-related intervention. The first concerns individuals, families, and systems *understanding* how to use best practice interventions. The second concerns the ability *to use* those interventions. Assistive technologies, or as we like to call them "cognitive prosthetics," are emerging that can help with both.

This chapter discusses several specific gaps that exist where *technology*, *health literacy*, and *health promotion* are not well coordinated today. We suggest a set of approaches at this interface where there is great potential for significant improvements in care delivery and outcomes. A brief review of the literature is provided to familiarize the reader with key concepts and advances to date. Health literacy interventions to improve outcomes are highlighted along with best practice approaches to health promotion. The application of current technology to enhance health promotion is provided to illustrate health literate interventions for a variety of populations. Application to older adults residing in rural communities is highlighted.

THE NEED FOR INCREASING ACCESS TO HEALTH CARE

Over the past decade, the National Institutes of Health and the National Science Foundation have increased the call for applications intended to advance scientific research and intervention regarding chronic illness, and HIV treatment adherence in particular. As the HIV epidemic has subsided, similar initiatives have been implemented for Alzheimer's disease and related dementias; heart disease has also been a focus, with a new emphasis on women's heart health. Three critical components can be identified in the scope of the policy initiative guiding these research initiatives:

1. Research is needed on novel, electronically mediated methods of delivering assessments and interventions to geographically or socially isolated populations.
2. Increased recognition of "prevention" as a key component of comprehensive health care is needed.
3. Treatment and adherence other than daily medication-taking behavior remains understudied and likely offers important contributions to patient care and health outcomes.

These policy initiatives and research directions are heavily influenced by the "Healthy People (HP) 2020" goals of improving quality and years of healthy life, and eliminating health disparities (www .healthypeople.gov). Disparity in health is related to disparity in access. Significant contributors to health care disparity include, among others, sociodemographic and socioeconomic factors, health insurance coverage and access to appropriate providers, and geographic region (Andrykowski, Steffens, Bush, & Tucker, 2014; Goris, Schutte, Rivard, & Schutte, 2015; Lefebvre & Metraux, 2009; Southwest Rural Health Research Center [SRHRC], n.d., http://sph.tamhsc.edu/srhrc/rhp2020.html).

RURAL INDIVIDUALS HAVE MORE BARRIERS TO HEALTH CARE AND HEALTH PROMOTION INTERVENTIONS

The underserved, particularly rural individuals, report inadequate access to health care and indicate a desire for health education and community-based programs to improve their health (Andrykowski et al., 2014; Bolin et al., 2015; Cudney, Weinert, & Kinion, 2011;

Martinez-Donate et al., 2013). Evidence suggests, when matched for gender and diagnosis, rural individuals are far worse off than their urban counterparts. They have trouble obtaining proper help with all major chronic illnesses including diabetes (Andrus, Kelly, Murphey, & Herndon, 2004; Wang, Balamuranugan, Biddle, & Rollins, 2011), mood and anxiety disorders, substance abuse (Andrykowski et al., 2014; Diala, Muntaner, & Walrath, 2004; Howell & McFeeters, 2008; McCulloch, Jackson, & Lassig, 2015), and intimate violence consequences (Anderson, Renner, & Bloom, 2014; Choo, Neward, Lowe, Hall, & McConnell, 2011; Logan, Walker, Cole, Ratliff, & Leukenfeld, 2003; Neill & Hammatt, 2015), and Multiple Sclerosis (Buchanan et al., 2006; Turner Chapko, Yanez, Leipertz, Whitham, Haselkorn, 2013).

Rural individuals, in particular, have significant challenges with respect to care; these challenges are well identified in "Rural HP 2020" (Bolin et al., 2015). Rural individuals and rural health care leaders list access to health care as their most important priority. This access includes services used to obtain care when an individual is ill and services available to promote health. Published research reviews and reports support these needs and priorities. However, reaching rural individuals in a health literate manner can be challenging.

Within the effort to achieve these goals comes the recognition of common factors influencing the health of individuals, communities, and the nation. Each identified health indicator in the 2020 HP documents relies in some part on what we would now label as health literacy:

- Information people have about their health and how to improve their health
- Choices people make that influence their overall health
- The context of where they live with respect to resources and constraints
- Adequate access to care (http://www.healthypeople.gov/LHI/Priorities.htm)

Primary issues, then, in the nation's effort to promote health become:

- How to develop health literate behaviorally focused interventions to increase knowledge of a healthy lifestyle
- How to best encourage the adoption and maintenance of behaviors identified as contributing to overall health
- How to reach the hard-to-reach individuals having limited access to care for a variety of reasons

LEVERAGING TECHNOLOGY OR eHEALTH TO IMPROVE ACCESS, ADHERENCE, AND ASSESSMENT

Some have espoused "eHealth" as one way to increase access and the potential advantages could be significant (Choi & Dinitto, 2013; Goris et al., 2015; Ritter, Robinette, & Cofano, 2010; Thorn, 2015; Watkins & Xie, 2014). Likely advantages include:

- Access to information tailored to an individual's needs
- Increased access to illness and wellness material previously limited to health care providers only
- Access of appropriate information at any time and place for healthy, ill, and disabled individuals
- Inclusion of special functions for those having visual, literacy, or disability issues
- Confidentiality with respect to obtaining information on highly sensitive health concerns

Smartphones and wireless technologies are changing the way our society lives and works. This emerging technology has found its way into many business niches. It has also had an impact on the health sciences in two unique ways: (a) it can foster enhanced connectivity to health care programs or providers and (b) it can be used to collect data in an individual's natural or real environment. Older handheld devices have been used to collect timed survey data from study participants and the data then returned to the researchers, a method known as "ecological momentary assessment" (EMA; Shifman, Stone, & Hufford, 2008). Smartphones have only just begun to be considered in a similar way to study health behaviors globally (Cho, Park, & Lee, 2014; Lo, Wu, Morra, Lee, & Reeves, 2012; Sterns, Sterns, Lax, Allen, & Hazelett, 2010).

Data collected with a handheld device, using EMA, is used in various ways. It can be matched to objective data such as pill counts gathered concurrently and reported to researchers. It can be compared to self-reported data collected retrospectively at intervals throughout a study. New wireless technologies can make gathering objective data more comfortable for study participants and smartphone technologies make possible real-time data collection and transfer within the context of an individual's daily life.

BENEFITS OF INCREASED ACCESS

Health-promoting interventions can improve outcomes for persons with a chronic illness and may be more successful when grounded in behavioral change theory. Rural individuals, in particular, have identified increased access to sick and well care, along with availability of appropriate health-oriented education, as key priorities. However, rural individuals living with chronic illness, especially older adults, report concerns in obtaining appropriate care given their limited community resources. Appropriate care includes accessible and health literate care. Delivering health-promoting interventions and assessing adherence to them using innovative technology such as an iPhone may be a cost-efficient and effective way to increase access to care and promote health for rural individuals. Such a method has the potential to address and define many of the unknown and unstudied questions related to living with chronic illness in rural settings.

eHEALTH HAS A HISTORY OF POSITIVE EDUCATIONAL IMPACTS ON RURAL INDIVIDUALS

The use of technology to address health-related issues in rural locations is not new. Hoolahan, Grosvenor, Kurtz, and Kelly (2007) found technology to enhance the ease of obtaining an increased understanding of health-related information. Heckman and Carlson (2007) used experimental methods and determined technology to be a supportive intervention with respect to decreasing health access barriers in rural individuals with HIV. Wathen and Harris (2007) qualitatively explored the use of technology to provide health-related information for rural women and found validation of the importance of e-resources when seeking health information. Caution, however, was expressed concerning health literacy and difficulty with accessing computer technology. Ritter and colleagues (2010) suggest a less-is-more approach with a recommendation to gain efficiencies utilizing concentrated telehealth centers rather than numerous smaller, less comprehensive satellite sites.

Healthy living guidelines provide a framework focusing on health, not illness (http://www.cdc.gov/healthyliving/). Healthy guidelines include multiple behaviors such as engaging in sufficient physical activity, maintaining a healthy diet, seeking preventative health services, and consistently making healthy choices, while avoiding risky behavior. Enhancing quality of life goals applies to those with minimal health issues as well as to those chronically ill or completely disabled. Individuals, however, must first know about healthy behaviors in order to use them.

THE HEALTHY BEHAVIOR OF EXCELLENT MEDICATION TAKING

Many chronic health conditions including heart disease, diabetes, and HIV require consistent, timely, and sustained adherence. Evidence-based practice guidelines for many conditions are readily available for clinicians (http://www.guideline.gov). These and other guidelines specify initiating and maintaining appropriate medications; however, there is evidence that among persons with chronic illness, health outcomes can also can be improved by using and adhering to other healthy behaviors (Abel, Hopson, & Delville, 2006; Antoni et al., 2006; Riley, Fava, Lewis, & Lewis, 2008; Sterns et al., 2010). Regardless, providing health literate information to those who need it most is not readily apparent in those guidelines. The degree to which preventative health behaviors are being used at optimum levels by individuals living with chronic illness needs to be better assessed. The structural barriers that exist for rural individuals, in particular, and that make challenging the reception of information about optimizing health outcomes with respect to living with a chronic illness need to be clearly identified and eliminated. Given the context of living in a rural environment where care access can be challenging, we need new approaches beyond the current paradigms commonly used by researchers to date.

INCORPORATING A HEALTH LITERACY COMPONENT INTO INTERVENTIONS

Research aimed at advancing the scientific understanding of chronic illness treatment should result in enhancing and expanding available intervention strategies for those with a chronic illness. We always encourage a health promotion component in the interventions we design (addressing multiple behaviors) using remote handheld computers ("smart" meaning Internet-connected devices). We have found that, particularly with rural individuals, we can thereby increase their access to health care services, enable and empower individuals' adoption and maintenance of and adherence to health-promoting behaviors, and support electronic assessment that can be used to establish and maintain positive health outcomes as a result of use of the technology-based intervention.

Health literacy programs have demonstrated improved treatment adherence with individuals (Bickmore et al., 2013; Gakumo, Enah, Vance, Sahinoglu, & Raper, 2015; Zulig, McCant, Melnyk, Danus, & Bosworth, 2014) and groups (Xie, 2011). But often, especially for older adults and assistive technology, interventions have inadequate consideration of health literacy, are atheoretical, and/or lack measurement of health outcomes (Watkins & Xie, 2014). Thus, the efficacy of using assistive technology to enhance health literacy and health outcomes is largely unknown.

THE HEALTH LITERACY AND HEALTH BEHAVIORAL CHALLENGE

Chronic Illness and Care Management

The use of cognitive prosthetics is contextualized within Wagner's chronic care model (CCM; Wagner, Austin, & Van Korff, 1996) and the medical traumatic stress processing model. Wagner and colleagues (1996) theorize that optimal care for patients with chronic illness is not possible in traditional health care systems that emphasize disease treatment over illness prevention because providers typically do not have the time, expertise, or data to provide the components required for effective chronic illness care. Medication adherence is a critical component of patient recovery and has proven particularly challenging to follow in real time in the community.

Nonadherence to Health-Promoting Behavior Is Expensive and Tragic

Since health promotion is viewed holistically, the detrimental effects of not using—or not adhering to—health promotion practices are similarly significant. Differential outcomes associated with use of healthy behaviors are well documented in the research literature (Nelson et al., 2015; Pinto & Schub, 2012; Takemura et al., 2011; Teri et al., 2011) including the impact of health literacy (Ahlers-Schmidt et al., 2012; Chin et al., 2015; Nelson et al., 2015; Zulig et al., 2014).

IDENTIFYING AND OVERCOMING BARRIERS TO TRAINING AND USAGE

The realization of the potential benefits of technology is dependent on the attitudes and usability needs of older adults. For instance, if one does not possess a positive attitude in the utility of learning to use such a device, the device is not likely to be adopted to assist medication adherence tasks, support education about the illness, or provide encouragement for positive behaviors such as exercise and good nutrition. Training and first exposure to new technology needs to be enticing, exciting, and fun.

In terms of the device itself, the hardware and software can both be barriers to receiving the benefits the device can deliver. As with early handheld devices, the screen displays were small and lacked the ability to display sharp contrasts compared to larger screens. In addition, the messages displayed and the controls are often small, making it more difficult to read and manipulate the interface. The hardware and software and the training to use them need to be carefully designed and tested (Sterns, 2005). We briefly describe the methods we have utilized to create a successful experience to overcome the barriers to realize the potential benefits of the proposed intervention and assessment technology.

Persuasive Software and Pillbox. To increase the number of people who can benefit from the long list of features a handheld computer can offer, the barriers to using the device must be addressed. Special usage skill training is required (Sterns, 2005) as well as creating software with improved interface and operation (Czaja & Lee, 2001) to improve the likelihood of success.

The most important design principle of an inviting and supporting medication adherence device is connecting instructions and information to the medication. The most serious drawback of plastic pillboxes is that they separate dosage and consumption instructions (e.g., take with water) and warnings (e.g., not to be taken with grapefruit juice) from medication.

To connect both together, an effective application will be capable of showing pictures of drugs so that the shape, color, and markings of the pills can be clearly seen. When looking at the details of a particular medication the name, dosage, number of tablets or capsules, and the reason for taking the pills must be presented. Contact information for the doctor, pharmacy, and a running pill count should also be featured. Finally, all buttons and text should be oversized for use by older adults. Sterns (2005) documents our initial software application called iRxReminder™ that provided all these features for a Palm OS-based device.

It is also important to link the reminder program and the medications. To accomplish this marriage, Sterns (2005) designed a patented pillbox attachment that integrates with a personal digital assistant or as we would refer to it today, a smartphone (see Figure 1). The pillbox case concept provides a way to carry midday medications or supplements. Sterns (2008) more recently proposed and received a patent for a smartphone case that integrates a pill container for carrying midday medications (see Figure 2). Ease-of-use and convenience

FIGURE 1 **The phone has a PalmOS-based app that provides support for medication tracking and reminding (left). The pillbox for carrying pills to be taken outside the home is mounted to the top of this early smartphone, a Samsung i300 (right).**

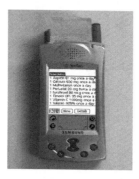
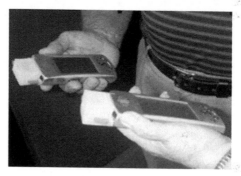

FIGURE 2 **These smartphone cases provide pill compartments to support midday medications. The smartphone, in this case an iPhone 4, utilizes the iRxReminder™ app to support medication tracking, reminding, and patient education.**

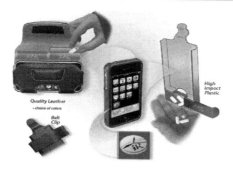

are essential elements to achieve the high adherence required for drug therapies for chronic illness.

ENHANCING HEALTH PROMOTION INTERVENTIONS USING TECHNOLOGY

We see the potential to more effectively and efficiently deliver health promotion recommendations beyond the physical clinical setting through utilizing the portable communication and media capabilities portable electronic devices provide. These devices will be ubiquitous for young, middle-aged, and young-older adults. For those older and oldest-old adults, there will be some who cannot benefit from interaction with these devices. This is true of every therapeutic approach; works for many, but not for all. We propose here establishing assessments and training that can be utilized to make these determinations. We believe handheld computers can provide the gateway to significant improvements in chronic care and health promotion programs specifically, and health generally.

Smart telecare and telemedicine intervention elements are delivered by specifically designed devices and through software running on a computer, on a smart device, or a combination. A model conceptual framework can be conceived where a computer-based intervention, a smartphone-based intervention, and specifically designed biometric and medication monitoring devices are all utilized together. When integrated, these interventions can deliver self- and family management intervention components. These components would improve the physical and psychological well-being of individuals and families recovering from an acute episode or living with a chronic condition. Such a model program might consist of a treatment consisting of a comprehensive patient self-management smartphone app, an online intervention support group, and an online web portal rich with information about accelerating recovery and highlighting caregiving resources. It might also include biometric monitoring devices such as a scale, pill dispensing hardware, and a digital activity monitor. All these activities could be coordinated by the platform's cloud component. When the person living with the chronic condition missed a regimen health behavior, the system would remind him or her. But importantly, if the behavior (e.g., weighing oneself, taking a pill) did occur, no nagging alert would be sounded. This avoids negative reinforcements through unnecessary nagging such as one gets from daily text reminders, and makes the alerts meaningful when the person really forgets. Thus, when the system is able to know the status of a person's behavior, it can be smart about reminding, thus, "cognitive prosthetic moniker."

One way to understand how an intervention operates is to consider it through the lens of the prominent stress processing model (Pearlin, Aneshensel, Mullan, & Whitlatch, 1995). The stress processing model is useful for identifying modifiable coping resources that affect the recovering individual and his or her caregiver's well-being, and examining how change in one model component may impact others. Past research gives evidence of the stress processing model's suitability to considering the impact on the individual and the caregiving dyad (Smith, Egbert, Dellman-Jenkins, Nanna, & Palmieri, 2012). According to the stress processing model (Pearlin, 2005), the stress process involves three core components: *stressors*, or demands and hardships that put physical and psychological capacities to test (e.g., recovery from an acute condition or having a chronic illness); *outcomes*, or the effects of stressors, including mental health and physical health; and *mediators*, the resources and behaviors that regulate how stressors affect outcomes. The resources of mastery, self-esteem, and social support consistently emerge as key factors that abate the adverse effects of stressors (Thoits, 2010). These stress processing model components account for sizeable variance in depression, and targeting interventions to enhance these resources ameliorates depression (Turner, Marino, & Rozell, 2003). Here we consider, at least qualitatively, the potential for technology-based interventions to act as a positive mediator that can improve mastery, self-esteem, and social support. We think of these as components of patient and family empowerment.

HEALTH ADHERENCE ASPECTS

Education

Patient education is one of the critical elements of successful chronic illness management. It can lead to increased participation in health promotion activities, may improve adherence to medical management recommendations (Bisset et al., 1997; Miller, Hill, Kottke, & Ockene, 1997), and is associated with positive outcomes such as decreased days in the hospital and decreased rehospitalizations. Following a chronic illness diagnosis, patient and family education may be especially critical since the recognition of and appropriate response to subsequent symptoms is a major determinant of patient outcomes (Pancioli et al., 1998).

A chronic disease care model is needed that emphasizes education to be healthier, exercise, eat well, and to improve patients' ability to recognize symptoms and their knowledge to seek appropriate medical attention at symptom onset (Pancioli et al., 1998; Sacco et al., 1997). Such a checklist could be presented in a booklet (as has been done by Allen et al., 2004) for another chronic illness, or on a handheld computer. The device can also be used to provide surveys of key symptoms at regular intervals and, if responses are problematic, respond appropriately (e.g., put up a message to call a doctor, send an alert to a relative, or send an alert to the primary care provide [PCP]). In this way, the device can serve a role in directing the device user to contact his or her care provider in a timely manner.

Medication Appropriateness and Adherence

In addition to providing education about medications, comprehensive care must address medication appropriateness and adherence. Many PCPs may be unaware of their patient's noncompliance, simply because no feedback on compliance is given to the provider. Thus, efforts to increase adherence with treatment should be incorporated into any comprehensive chronic care management model.

Another medication issue is suboptimal prescribing. An inappropriate medication regimen includes drugs associated with excessive risk of renal damage, bleeding, falls, cognitive impairment, incontinence, and diminished cardiovascular, gastrointestinal, and pulmonary health. Also, an inappropriate drug regimen might fail to include state-of-the-art, evidence-based medications for cardiovascular problems, and medications to treat the common complication of depression. Finally, patients may be on several medications associated with serious multi-drug interactions. Hanlon and Artz (2001) refer to such prescribing practices as a major health issue that leads to significant morbidity and mortality. They cite evidence that multidisciplinary teams can be effective in reducing the problem of suboptimal prescribing. Utilizing the PDA to collect all prescriptions, supplements, and OTC medications and assessment for appropriateness (first by the research team and later by the PCP) should eliminate suboptimal prescribing. Further information about adherence, mood, and impacts on instrumental activities of daily living will enhance the PCP's ability to tune the dosages and time of day the medications are taken.

PHYSICAL MEASURES OF HEALTH

Blood Pressure and Cholesterol Control

As individuals living with chronic illness live longer, they will be increasingly affected by health issues affecting aging individuals, particularly hypertension and high cholesterol. The PDA can remind people to get their pressure checked and provide a place to record the blood pressure. Devices will be available in the third quarter of 2008 that can take blood pressure, glucose levels, and EKG from the arm and send the results via BlueTooth to the PDA. The data can be shared with a doctor. A PDA can help control cholesterol by improving medication taking, reordering, and ensuring appointments are kept for monitoring levels. PDA delivers reminders about blood pressure checks at local pharmacies and, utilizing wireless equipment, can collect and summarize the data for review at the PCP exam. Unusual or out-of-range readings can trigger a contact right on the phone with a care manager who can recommend further action.

Exercise

Physical inactivity is a major risk factor for cardiovascular disease (NIH Consensus Development Panel on Physical Activity and Cardiovascular Health, 1996). An increased level of physical activity is known to affect overall health, mood, and function. The Joint National Committee on Prevention, Evaluation and Treatment of Hypertension (1997) recommends increased levels of physical activity to help control blood pressure. Regular surveys about the amount of exercise can serve as a trigger for increasing exercise and provide important data during examinations with the PCP.

SUMMARY OF PROPOSED BENEFITS FROM COGNITIVE PROSTHETICS FOR HEALTH PROMOTION

Treating chronic illness is expensive and challenging considering individual, community, and national costs. The medications themselves can be expensive; not properly taking medications can be even more expensive with respect to viral resistance and health outcomes. Adherence to a health-promoting lifestyle has the potential to enhance individuals' general health and improve their ability to live a life not dictated by their illness. Improved self-management is now possible with handheld electronic devices. These devices can be successful because they have communication features that make the device likely to be carried by the individual. Sterns (2005) and Sterns and Mayhorn (2006) have shown that individuals with chronic illness and minimal mobile computing experience can, and will, embrace handheld computers and use them successfully for voice communication, e-mail, tracking contacts and appointments, responding to surveys, and improving medication adherence. Of the new generation of smartphones, recent models with their touch interface, large bright screens, and no small buttons for input, provide the best commercial platform yet for ease-of-use, particularly with middle-aged adults and older. Android and iOS have publicly available development programs to allow commercial development of software and provide virtual stores (e.g., App Store) for distribution.

The electronic platform can support improved health promotion, particularly aspects important to individuals living with chronic illness. Most importantly, medication adherence can be managed and recorded. Short audio and video educational presentations utilizing the podcast media features can provide individuals with the information necessary to learn more about promoting health within their chronic illness. Survey questions can be used intermittently to detect ongoing adherence to the behaviors and collect data on other information related to a person's prescription and overall wellness. This data can be sent in real time from the field to a monitoring computer supported by a health care team member who can respond to triggered alerts; immediately when urgent, and more slowly when not. In the future it could also be summarized and added to the electronic medical record of a patient to support evaluation and ongoing treatment by the primary care physician and other specialists. It is certain that such a system will help stretch the finite resources as the global population ages.

REFERENCES

Abel, E., Hopson, L., & Delville, C. (2006). Health promotion for women with human immunodeficiency virus or acquired immunodeficiency syndrome. *Journal of the American Academy of Nurse Practitioners, 18*, 534–543. Retrieved from http://search.ebscohost.com/login.aspx?direct=true&db=cmedm&AN=17064331&site=ehost-live

Ahlers-Schmidt, C., Chesser, A. K., Paschal, A. M., Hart, T. A., Williams, K. S., Yaghmai, B., & Shah-Haque, S. (2012). Parent opinions about use of text messaging for immunization reminders. *Journal of Medical Internet Research, 14*(3), e83–e83. Retrieved from http://ezproxy.uakron.edu:2048/login?url=http://search.ebsco-host.com/login.aspx?direct=true&db=rzh&AN=2011643911&site=ehost-live

Allen, K. R., Hazelett, S., Jarjora, D., Wright, K., Clough, L., & Weinhardt, J. (2004). Improving stroke outcomes: Implementation of a post-discharge care management model. *Chronic Care, 11*, 707–714.

Anderson, K. M., Renner, L. M., & Bloom, T. S. (2014). Rural women's strategic responses to intimate partner violence. *Health Care for Women International, 35*(4), 423–441. doi:10.1080/07399332.2013.815757

Andrus, M. R., Kelley, K. W., Murphey, L. M., & Herndon, K. C. (2004). A comparison of diabetes care in rural and urban medical clinics in Alabama. *Journal of Community Health, 29*(1), 29–44.

Andrykowski, M. A., Steffens, R. F., Bush, H. M., & Tucker, T. C. (2014). Disparities in mental health outcomes among lung cancer survivors associated with ruralness of residence. *Psycho-Oncology, 23*(4), 428–436. doi:10.1002/pon.3440

Antoni, M. H., Lechner, S. C., Kazi, A., Wimberly, S. R., Sifre, T., Urcuyo, K. R., . . . Carver, C. S. (2006). How stress management improves quality of life after treatment for breast cancer. *Journal of Consulting and Clinical Psychology, 74*, 1143–1152.

Bickmore, T. W., Silliman, R. A., Nelson, K., Cheng, D. M., Winter, M., Henault, L., & Paasche-Orlow, M. (2013). A randomized controlled trial of an automated exercise coach for older adults. *Journal of the American Geriatrics Society, 61*(10), 1676-1683. doi:10.1111/jgs.12449

Bisset, A., MacDuff, C., Chesson, R., & Maitland, J. (1997). Stroke services in general practice—Are they satisfactory?. *British Journal of General Practice, 47*, 787–793.

Bolin, J. N., Bellamy, G. R., Ferdinand, A. O., Vuong, A. M., Kash, B. A., Schulze, A., & Helduser, J. W. (2015). Rural healthy people 2020: New decade, same challenges. *Journal of Rural Health: Official Journal of the American Rural Health Association and the National Rural Health Care Association, 31*(3), 326–333. doi:10.1111/jrh.12116

Buchanan, R. J., Stuifbergen, A., Chakravorty, B. J., Wang, S., Zhu, L., & Kim, M. (2006). Urban/rural differences in access and barriers to health care for people with multiple sclerosis. *Journal of Health and Human Services Administration, 29*, 360–375. Retrieved from http://search.ebscohost.com/login.aspx?direct=true&db=cmedm&AN=17571473&site=ehost-live

CDC. (2015). *Guidelines and recommendations*. Retreived from http://www.cdc.gov/hiv/guidelines

Chin, J., Madison, A., Gao, X., Graumlich, J. F., Conner-Garcia, T., Murray, M. D., . . . Morrow, D. G. (2015). Cognition and health literacy in older adults' recall of self-care information. *Gerontologist*. Retrieved from http://ezproxy.uakron.edu:2048/login?url=http://search.ebscohost.com/login.aspx?direct=true&db=mnh&AN=26209450&site=ehost-live

Cho, J., Park, D., & Lee, H. E. (2014). Cognitive factors of using health apps: Systematic analysis of relationships among health consciousness, health information orientation, eHealth literacy, and health app use efficacy. *Journal of Medical Internet Research, 16*(5), e125–e125. doi:10.2196/jmir.3283

Choi, N. G., & Dinitto, D. M. (2013). The digital divide among low-income homebound older adults: Internet use patterns, eHealth literacy, and attitudes toward computer/Internet use. *Journal of Medical Internet Research, 15*(5), e93. doi:10.2196/jmir.2645

Choo, E. K., Newgard, C. D., Lowe, R. A., Hall, M. K., & McConnell, K. J. (2011). Rural-urban disparities in emergency department intimate partner violence resources. *Western Journal of Emergency Medicine: Integrating Emergency Care With Population Health, 12*(2), 178–183. Retrieved from http:// ezproxy.uakron.edu:2048/login?url=http://search.ebscohost.com/login .aspx?direct=true&db=rzh&AN=2011058949&site=ehost-live

Cudney, S., Weinert, C., & Kinion, E. (2011). Forging partnerships between rural women with chronic conditions and their health care providers. *Journal of Holistic Nursing: Official Journal of the American Holistic Nurses' Association, 29*(1), 53–60. doi:10.1177/0898010110373656

Czaja, S. J., & Lee, C. C. (2001). The Internet and older adults: Design challenges and opportunities. In N. Charness & D. Park (Eds.), *Communication, technology, and aging: Opportunities and challenges for the future* (pp. 60–78). New York, NY: Springer Publishing.

Diala, C. C., Muntaner, C., & Walrath, C. (2004). Gender, occupational, and socioeconomic correlates of alcohol and drug abuse among U.S. rural, metropolitan, and urban residents. *American Journal of Drug and Alcohol Abuse, 30,* 409–428. Retrieved from http://search.ebscohost.com/login .aspx?direct=true&db=cmedm&AN=15230083&site=ehost-live

Gakumo, C. A., Enah, C. C., Vance, D. E., Sahinoglu, E., & Raper, J. L. (2015). "Keep it simple": Older African Americans' preferences for a health literacy intervention in HIV management. *Patient Preference and Adherence, 9,* 217–223. doi:10.2147/ PPA.S69763

Goris, E. D., Schutte, D. L., Rivard, J. L., & Schutte, B. C. (2015). Community leader perceptions of the health needs of older adults. *Western Journal of Nursing Research, 37*(5), 599–618. doi:10.1177/0193945914530046

Hanlon, J. T., & Artz, M. B. (2001). Drug-related problems and pharmaceutical care: What are they, do they matter, and what's next? *Medical Care, 39*(2), 109–112.

Heckman, T. G., & Carlson, B. (2007). A randomized clinical trial of two telephone-delivered, mental health interventions for HIV-infected persons in rural areas of the United States. *AIDS and Behavior, 11*(1), 5–14.

Hoolahan, B., Grosvenor, J., Kurtz, H., & Kelly, B. (2007). Utilizing technology to raise mental health literacy in small rural towns. *Learning in Health and Social Care, 6*(3), 145–155.

Howell, E., & McFeeters, J. (2008). Children's mental health care: Differences by race/ethnicity in urban/rural areas. *Journal of Health Care for the Poor and Underserved, 19*(1), 237–247. Retrieved from http://search.ebscohost.com/login .aspx?direct=true&db=rzh&AN=2009812396&site=ehost-live

Lefebvre, K. M., & Metraux, S. (2009). Disparities in level of amputation among minorities: Implications for improved preventative care. *Journal of the National Medical Association, 101*(7), 649–655. Retrieved from http://search.ebscohost.com/login .aspx?direct=true&db=rzh&AN=2010354705&site=ehost-live

Lo, V., Wu, R. C., Morra, D., Lee, L., & Reeves, S. (2012). The use of smartphones in general and internal medicine units: A boon or a bane to the promotion of interprofessional collaboration? *Journal of Interprofessional Care, 26*(4), 276–282. doi:10.3109/13561820.2012.663013

Logan, T. K., Walker, R., Cole, J., Ratliff, S., & Leukefeld, C. (2003). Qualitative differences among rural and urban intimate violence victimization experiences and consequences: A pilot study. *Journal of Family Violence, 18,* 83–92. Retrieved from http://search.ebscohost.com/login .aspx?direct=true&db=rzh&AN=2004154870&site=ehost-live

Martinez-Donate, A., Halverson, J., Simon, N., Strickland, J. S., Trentham-Dietz, A., Smith, P. D., . . . Wang, X. (2013). Identifying health literacy and health system navigation needs among rural cancer patients: Findings from the rural oncology literacy enhancement study (ROLES). *Journal of Cancer Education, 28*(3), 573–581. doi:10.1007/s13187-013-0505-x

McCulloch, B. J., Jackson, M. N. G., & Lassig, S. L. (2015). Worry and bother: Factors in rural women's health decision making. *Journal of Women and Aging, 27*(3), 251–265. doi:10.1080/08952841.2014.934645

Miller, N. H., Hill, M., Kottke, T., & Ockene, I. S. (1997). The multilevel compliance challenge: Recommendations for a call to action. A statement for healthcare professionals. *Circulation, 95*(4), 1085–1090.

Neill, K. S., & Hammatt, J. (2015). Beyond urban places: Responding to intimate partner violence in rural and remote areas. *Journal of Forensic Nursing, 11*(2), 93–100. doi:10.1097/JFN.0000000000000070

Nelson, L. A., Mulvaney, S. A., Gebretsadik, T., Ho, Y., Johnson, K. B., & Osborn, C. Y. (2015). Disparities in the use of a mHealth medication adherence promotion intervention for low-income adults with type 2 diabetes. *Journal of the American Medical Informatics Association, 23*(1), 12–18. doi:10.1093/jamia/ocv082

Pancioli, A., Broderick, J., Kothari, R., Brott, T., Tuchfarber, A., Miller, R., . . . Jauch, E. (1998). Public perception of stroke warning signs and knowledge of potential risk factors. *Journal of the American Medical Association, 279*(16), 1288–1292.

Park, D. C., & Jones, T. R. (1997). Medication adherence and aging. In A. D. Fisk & A. Rogers (Eds.), *Handbook of human factors and the older adult* (p. 257). Mahwah, NJ: Lawrence Erlbaum.

Pearlin, L. I. (2005). In A. Maney & J. Ramos (Eds.), Some conceptual perspectives on the origins and prevention of social stress. *Socioeconomic conditions, stress and mental disorders: Toward a new synthesis of research and public policy.* Retrieved from http://www.mhsip.org, Mental Health Statistics Program Online. pp. 1–35.

Pearlin, L. I., Aneshensel, C. S., Mullan, J. T., & Whitlatch, C. J. (1995). Caregiving and its social support. In L. K. George, & R. H. Binstock (Eds.), *Handbook of aging and the social sciences* (4th ed., pp. 283–302). San Diego, CA: Academic Press.

Pinto, S., & Schub, T. (2012). In D. Pravikoff & D. Pravikoff (Eds.), *Patient adherence to medical treatment: The effect of social support.* Glendale, CA: Cinahl Information Systems. Retrieved from http://search.ebscohost.com/login .aspx?direct=true&db=rzh&AN=5000001140&site=ehost-live

Riley, T. A., Lewis, B. M., Lewis, M. P., & Fava, J. L. (2008). Low-income HIV-infected women and the process of engaging in healthy behavior. *Journal of Association of Nurses in AIDS Care, 9,* 3–15. Retrieved from http://search.ebscohost.com/login .aspx?direct=true&db=rzh&AN=2009770465&site=ehost-live

Ritter, L. A., Robinette, T. R., & Cofano, J. (2010). Evaluation of a statewide telemedicine program. *Californian Journal of Health Promotion, 8*(1), 1–9. Retrieved from http://search.ebscohost.com/login.aspx?direct=true&db=rzh&AN=201 0910003&site=ehost-live

Sacco, R. L., Benjamin, E. J., Broderick, J. P., Dyken, M., Easton, J. D., Feinberg, W. M., . . . Wolf, P. A. (1997). Risk factors. *Stroke, 28,* 1507–1517.

Smith, G. C., Egbert, N., Dellman-Jenkins, M., Nanna, K., & Palmieri, P. A. (2012). Reducing depression in stroke survivors and their informal caregivers: A randomized clinical trial of a web-based intervention. *Rehabilitation Psychology, 57*(3), 196–206. PMCID:3434961

Southwest Rural Health Research Center. (n.d.). *Rural healthy people 2010.* Retrieved from http://www.srph.tamhsc.edu/centers/rhp2010/introvol1.htm

Sterns, A. (2005). Curriculum design and program to train older adults to use personal digital assistants. *Gerontologist, 45*(6), 828–834.

Sterns, A. A., Lax, G., Sterns, H., Allen, K., & Hazelet, S. (2010, May). Improving chronic care management: An iPhone application for post-stroke recovery. Paper delivered at the International Society of Gerontechnology conference in Vancouver, BC, Canada.

Sterns, A. A., & Mayhorn, C. B. (2006). Persuasive pillboxes: Improving medication adherence with personal digital assistants. In Y. de Kort & W. I. Jsselsteijn (Eds.), *Persuasive technologies.* New York, NY: Springer Publishing.

Takemura, M., Mitsui, K., Itotani, R., Ishitoko, M., Suzuki, S., Matsumoto, M., . . . Fukui, M. (2011). Relationships between repeated instruction on inhalation therapy, medication adherence, and health status in chronic obstructive pulmonary disease. *International Journal of Chronic Obstructive Pulmonary Disease, 6,* 97–104. Retrieved from http://search.ebscohost.com/login .aspx?direct=true&db=mnh&AN=21407822&site=ehost-live

Teri, L., McCurry, S. M., Logsdon, R. G., Gibbons, L. E., Buchner, D. M., & Larson, E. B. (2011). A randomized controlled clinical trial of the Seattle protocol for activity in older adults. *Journal of the American Geriatrics Society, 59*(7), 1188–1196. doi:10.1111/j.1532-5415.2011.03454.x

Thoits, P. A. (2010). Stress and health: Major findings and policy implications. *Journal of Health and Social Behavior, 51*(Supplement 1), S41–S53.

Turner, A. P., Chapko, M. K., Yanez, D., Leipertz, S. L., Sloan, A. P., Whitham, R. H., & Haselkorn, J. K. (2013). Access to multiple sclerosis specialty care. *PM&R, 5*(12), 1044–1050. doi:10.1016/j.pmrj.2013.07.009

Turner, R. J., Marino, F., & Rozell, P. (2003). On the stress process as mechanism in the social distribution of mental disease: Community studies. *Socioeconomic conditions, stress and mental disorders: Toward a new synthesis of research and public policy* (pp. 1–34). Retrieved from http://www.mhsip.org, Mental Health Statistics Program Online.

Wagner, E., Austin, B., & Von Korff, M. (1996). Organizing care for patients with chronic illness. *Millbank Quarterly, 74*(4), 511–544.

Wang, W., Balamurugan, A., Biddle, J., & Rollins, K. M. (2011). Diabetic neuropathy status and the concerns in underserved rural communities: Challenges and opportunities for diabetes educators. *Diabetes Educator, 37*(4), 536–548. doi:10.1177/0145721711410717

Wathen, C. N., & Harris, R. M. (2007). "I try to take care of it myself." How rural women search for health information. *Qualitative Health Research, 17*(5), 639–651.

Watkins, I., & Xie, B. (2014). eHealth literacy interventions for older adults: A systematic review of the literature. *Journal of Medical Internet Research, 16*(11), e225–e225. doi:10.2196/jmir.3318

Xie, B. (2011). Effects of an eHealth literacy intervention for older adults. *Journal of Medical Internet Research, 13*(4), e90. doi:10.2196/jmir.1880

CHAPTER 11

Gold Standard Programs to Assist Older Adults in Healthier Living

THERESA B. SKAAR, TARA P. MCCOY, AND KERRY S. KLEYMAN

In the documentary *Alive Inside*, Rossato-Bennett explores how music revitalizes and awakens older individuals across the country. Music carves a path to youthfulness and is an inspiration that makes us happy; he states, "there is no pill that does that" (Rossato-Bennett, 2014). The documentary centers on a nonprofit organization called Music & Memory, which provides older adults with the therapeutic benefits of personalized music (i.e., playlists of music that has impacted their lives across their life spans), and is a fast-growing evidence-based program using music to improve quality of life for older adults.

> Music has more ability to activate more parts of the brain than any other stimulus . . . by exciting or awakening those pathways, we have a gateway to stimulate and reach somebody who is otherwise unreachable.
>
> *(Rossato-Bennett, 2014)*

What is most striking about the Music & Memory program is the simplicity of the idea. It first launched as an idea based on the research of neurologist, Oliver Saks, who asked the question, "Why do musical memories linger long after other memories have faded?" This program offers adults in late adulthood access to music by providing them with donated iPods and mp3 players with music tailored to their liking (i.e., from their formative years). This simple intervention can help increase positive feelings through nostalgic reminiscing. When something as simple and inexpensive as a donated iPod can be used to create a calmer, supportive environment, leading to residents who are happier and more social, the question then begs, what other inexpensive programming can be created to increase the overall quality of life?

In this chapter, we explore some of the primary problems that plague the older adult population, such as dehydration, and discuss how these problems are related to and may be remedied by increasing health literacy (one's ability to understand and obtain necessary information regarding their health care). Additionally, we outline our suggestions for various low-cost environmental interventions, such as music implementation and educational programs that may help promote healthier living among older adult populations.

WHAT IS HEALTH LITERACY?

"Health literacy" as defined by the World Health Organization (World Health Organization, 1998) is "the cognitive and social skills which determine the motivation and ability of individuals to gain access to, understand, and use information in ways which promote and maintain good health." In other words, it is considered to be individuals' ability to acquire and comprehend health information and to ultimately act in accordance with said information. One example of health literacy includes knowing where to look for information, such as on a prescription bottle or knowing how many pills to take in a day (Rudd, 2007). "Literacy," similar to health literacy, is generally defined as individuals' ability to read and understand information in many contexts, one of which could include health care.

General literacy skills are an important component of health literacy (Ishikawa & Yano, 2008). If one lacks the ability to read, it is very difficult for him or her to follow directions, such as those listed on a prescription bottle. It should be noted, however, that literacy skills can be domain specific; therefore, having high literacy skills in general (i.e., high reading comprehension) may not always transfer to the health domain (Ratzan & Parker, 2006). Consider the following example: Jane, a 72-year-old adult, has great reading abilities. She is prescribed to take two tablespoons of medication, two times per day. However, because her standard dosing cup is labeled only in milliliters (mL), she assumes two capfuls (60 mL) are equivalent to her necessary dosage. This leads Jane to take two times the amount of medication needed for a given day. Jane's general literacy skills were not enough for her to adhere to her health plan properly due to lack of knowledge as to where additional necessary information could be obtained; demonstrating that she lacked the necessary health literacy skills. Errors such as this can lead to serious health implications, especially considering the amount of medication some individuals may need to consume in a single day.

The Importance of Health Literacy in Older Adult Populations

In a 2003 national survey, 59% of Americans 65 years of age or older were found to have basic or below basic levels of health literacy (Kutner, Greenburg, Jin, & Paulsen, 2006). Older adults had the lowest levels of intermediate and proficient health literacy compared to all other age groups. This is alarming considering that individuals at an intermediate level of health literacy are able to "determine what time a person can take a prescription medication, based on information on the prescription drug label that relates the timing of medication to eating" (p. 6). Creating interventions for increasing health literacy in older adults is necessary in order to inform a majority of this population of the very rudimentary tasks involved in medication adherence.

Given this information, it should come as no surprise that health literacy is related to various outcomes that may, in turn, influence how well individuals are able to function within a health context. When people have difficulty comprehending the information they are given pertaining to their health, some of their health outcomes may falter. Health literacy is, arguably, more important for older adults who have greater health care needs. **Chronic conditions** (illnesses persisting for a long period of time) tend to become more prevalent in late adulthood (Moody & Sasser, 2015). Chronic conditions often require medical intervention, therefore if an individual has low health literacy skills they might have difficulty following the prescribed treatment plan. For example, in the United States, approximately 25% of adults aged 65 or older have diabetes (Centers for Disease Control and Prevention, 2014). Poor health literacy has been found to be predictive of worse glycemic control and an increased frequency of retinopathy in individuals with type 2 diabetes (Schillinger et al., 2002). This information, taken together, suggests that older individuals may be at greater risk for complications with their diabetes control. Although there are several interventions that can treat diabetes (e.g., glycemic control), without health literacy skills, it is unlikely that the interventions will be effective.

In sum, older adults are at an increased risk for health deficits such as dehydration and general nutritional deficiencies. These problems may become intensified when individuals lack health literacy skills. Therefore, it is essential to understand how health literacy specifically impacts older populations and how these impacts can be decreased through health literacy interventions.

THE NATURE OF THE PROBLEM

Health literacy is undoubtedly an important tool to have in one's "kit." It provides individuals with the necessary skills and information needed to understand and process the information exchanged with their health care providers. Unfortunately, the state of health care with older adult populations is far more complex. The following focus on the current state and challenges facing health care and health care providers.

The State of Health Care Providers and Older Adult Populations

In previous generations, it was common practice for adult children to be responsible for the care of their aging parents. Over the past half century, these familial obligations and norms have shifted dramatically due to an increase in longevity, changes in family structure, and more women in the workforce (Hofstede, 1980; Moody & Sasser, 2015). Due to these and other societal changes, many families today rely on external means such as independent and assisted living facilities to provide support for their aging family members. For example, in 2012, approximately 8 million people in the United States utilized the services of about 58,500 regulated long-term care services (Harris-Kojetin, Sengupta, Park-Lee, & Valverde, 2013), and this number continues to grow as the baby boomer population begins to phase into retirement.

"Long-term care services" identified by the Centers for Disease Control and Prevention (2013) include adult day service centers, home health agencies, hospices, nursing homes, and similar residential care communities. The need for long-term services has increased significantly over the past few decades. Ribbe and colleagues (1997) used data from 1993 to report that the United States had approximately 2,100 nursing homes serving 1.5 million elder residents. The trend of "aging migration" (elders transitioning from residing independently to communal living, oftentimes with medical and personal care assistance) shows the increasing need for a focus on health and health care in these specific contexts.

Furthermore, this shift has been influential in the way in which health information is disseminated. Essentially, there is a gap in the communication process between **health care providers** (people who help in identifying or preventing or treating illness or disability) and patients. First, the large number of older adults requiring care creates a deficit in the *patient–provider ratio* (individuals needing care and the number of providers available to give that care), which in turn leads to limited resources (e.g., staff, time; higher patient turnover increases in severity of illness, health care provider staff is not increased to match the level of care needed; Welton, 2007). Per the U.S. Department of Health and Human Services (U.S. Department of Health and Human Services, 2014), this deficit continues to expand as the largest aging population, the baby boomer generation, enters into and beyond retirement.

Given this information, the challenge is to create sustainable programs that are realistic for health care workers to implement and accessible to all levels and budgets within their systems. However, currently there is a substantial lack of evidence-based, simple, and low-cost programs that would fit into this skewed patient–provider environment. According to the CDC, evidence-based programs must meet the following criteria: (a) evaluation research can produce the hypothesized positive results, (b) the results have strong internal validity, (c) the research goes through the peer review process, and (d) the program is endorsed by a federal agency or research organization (Spencer et al., 2013).

Moreover, with an increase in patient workloads and (over) reliance on technologies, communication issues remain a persistent challenge between patient and provider. Weiss and Blustein (1996) found that patients who maintained long-term relationships with their physicians tended to have lower costs of inpatient and outpatient care, including a reduction in hospitalizations. Patients also tend to report greater satisfaction when they believe that they have their physician's support when making health-related decisions (Dugdale, Epstein, & Pantilat, 1999). This evidence suggests that it is critical for patients and providers to have effective communication. However, despite the benefits of physician–patient relationships, this level of personal care and attention is a challenge for providers to offer. For instance, the amount of time a physician spends with a patient during a typical visit has decreased drastically over the years, averaging approximately 11 to 15 minutes today (Rabin, 2014), compared to 20 to 26 minutes in 1993 (Dugdale et al., 1999).

In this "connected" era (information accessible online), providers may also have expectations that their clients have done some footwork ahead of time. This, however, may not be the case for the older adult population. This suggests a disconnect occurring between the information necessary for elders to understand their own health care needs and their treatment plans (i.e., they lack the knowledge and accessibility to promote their own success). With a reliance on technology and more tech-savvy younger patients, the elders without the technological skills and experience simply lack the tools to stay abreast of the rapidly changing medical and health information available. The generational differences in self-efficacy relating to health care (i.e., the belief in one's ability to understand and manage health care) create a barrier to the largest group of health care consumers, elders. As such, developing alternative modes of education, availability, and efficacy in this population through evidence-based programming is essential (Frosch & Elwyn, 2014).

Finally, the high occurrence of comorbidity (simultaneous presence of two chronic diseases or conditions in a patient) in elders living in assisted oriented facilities presents another challenge. These health issues may range from cognitive deficiencies (e.g., Alzheimer's disease) to psychological disturbances (e.g., depression) to physical ailments (e.g., inability to walk). Some of these health issues have the potential to be remedied or, at the very least, improved. Research has shown that with simple interventions, and increases in health literacy, elders can live more fulfilling and satisfying lives (Moody & Sasser, 2015). Thus, it is imperative to consider the variation in elders' abilities to engage in and understand health interventions, creating a need for flexible strategies to effectively involve people at all levels of health literacy (Frosch & Elwyn, 2014).

As evidenced here, there are several potential challenges in creating programs to increase health behaviors and literacy in the elder population. Challenges include limited resources (e.g. health care workers tend to have large caseloads), communication difficulties between health care providers and patients, and high occurrences of comorbidity in elder patients. Many of these challenges can be addressed by assisting elders to become more active (rather than passive) patients. By developing health care literacy, health efficacy, and accessible educational tools, today's aging adults can be more proactive in their own health. Regarding the changes in health care over the years and limited traditional resources (e.g., direct family involvement, time availability of health professionals), it is important to find creative solutions to assist elders in integrating new behaviors that encourage healthier living; and further, there is the need to disseminate life-improving health information to elders in a proactive and meaningful way.

The Challenges to Health Care Providers

Consider the following scenario: A certified nursing assistant (CNA) is tasked with the responsibility to tend to an entire floor of older adult individuals, all with differing mental and physical limitations. During a typical shift, the CNA is required to provide the patients on this floor with their daily medication regime, assist with hygiene needs (e.g., bathing), and complete necessary paperwork. Given that no one else is there to help, the CNA does not have the ability, due to time restraints, to discuss a patient's questions or concerns regarding alternative medication options, or other health-related questions. Instead, the CNA provides the patient with a list of websites for the patient to search. The patient, unfortunately, does not have the necessary computer skills to find the information. This leaves the patient confused, unsure how to proceed regarding his or her health, and unsure of where to turn. It is important to keep in mind that scenarios such as this are not uncommon, as many health care providers, as mentioned, tend to have far more patients than they have time for.

The aforementioned scenario does not only depict an example of health care workers' time constraints, it also showcases another common problem in older adult populations, and that is, as mentioned previously, health literacy. The underlying question is: How can older adults become more health literate?

In most cases, older adults become more literate through educational programs in their living facilities and from their interactions with their physicians and health care providers. However, the problem within this domain is that health literacy is not health care workers' primary objective during their daily routines; and in fact, in most cases, it simply is not on their radar at all. Further, health care professionals may feel overburdened due to limited time with patients as well as demands due to increases in paperwork (Chen, 2013) and may be unwilling to take on another program to disseminate information. Thus, assisting older adults in obtaining higher levels of health literacy may feel taxing to health care professionals. For example, many interventions (relating to health literacy as well as direct care) are centered on staff involvement, such as requiring staff to provide direct and consistent prompts (i.e., every 1.5 hours) to increase hydration in nursing home residents (Feliciano, LeBlanc, & Feeney, 2010; Spangler, Risley, & Bilyew, 1984). Given the number of patients a health care provider might be charged with each shift, it is important to consider the limitations of the health care system in sustaining programs when developing interventions and to design them in such a way as to be easily maintained after grant support for the study ends (Frosch & Elwyn, 2014).

For most of us, it is hard to imagine that someone else may know more about us than ourselves. We fall prey to the "false consensus effect," overestimating that if we know something, everyone else probably does as well (Ross, Greene, & House, 1977). This sets the stage for understanding the perspective of the health care provider. It is not unusual for health care providers to perceive a lack of health literacy as a deficit with the patient (Frosch & Elwyn, 2014). This, in turn, can lead to frustration in the interactions between the provider and patient. For example, a CNA may become frustrated that the patient doesn't understand his or her medical condition, causing the CNA to treat the patient in a childish manner. On the flip side, the patient, wanting to ask questions, is reluctant to ask them due to the negative attitude and childish treatment by the CNA, causing the patient to simply nod and not gain any new information. This type of cyclical communication is an example of self-fulfilling prophecy, which indicates individuals' behaviors will change to become consistent with another person's expectations (Rosenthal & Jacobson, 1968). Specifically, if health care workers expect patients to simply comply with directions and not ask questions, then that is likely to be the behavior they will engage in.

Negative interactions, such as those suggested earlier, may decrease health care professionals' willingness to lead or participate in programs designed to increase health literacy in older adults. Additionally, it may decrease the willingness of the patients. This is evidenced by studies suggesting that patients are concerned that if they ask questions, they will be perceived as difficult or demanding (Frosch & Elwyn, 2014). It is important for older adults to feel comfortable asking questions and engaging in conversation with health care providers in order for them to obtain optimal health and health care. But it is also imperative to create programs and interventions that will: (a) decrease negative communication interactions, (b) be easy to implement and be timesaving, and (c) create a safe and positive environment for both provider and patient.

Today's older adult population is much less homogeneous than typically portrayed, with differences in social and cultural backgrounds, varying degrees of cognitive and physical abilities, and increased differences in language and literacy (Moody & Sasser, 2015). Thus, it is impractical to think that health care providers have all of the information necessary to guide and direct each individual patient. Therefore, the focus on programming should focus on simple programs that increase positive communication, decrease interaction biases, and are low-cost/low-effort for the provider. In the next sections, we focus on defining health literacy through some common examples of prevalent issues in older generations, such as dehydration.

THEORETICAL MODELS TO ENGAGE IN HEALTHY LIVING

The primary goal in this endeavor is to promote healthy living through evidence-based programming. There are many components to a person's ability to engage in healthy behavior, from differing motivations to individual differences. However, the current section focuses on a model that brings together many of these components to create a more usable model in designing programming, and that is the Theory of Planned Behavior (TPB).

Theory of Planned Behavior

One of the goals of health literacy, not surprisingly, is to increase healthy behaviors. Changing behaviors, especially ones that have been habituated for several decades, is not an easy task. For illustration, individuals who have been able to remain relatively healthy without completely adhering to medical regimens (e.g., prescription drugs) during earlier years of life may be more reluctant to strictly adhere to their medications as older adults. However, health literacy interventions need to address the behavioral components of individuals' health beyond offering them the skills to access and understand their health information (cognitive components). Based on this example, we can begin to understand how the TPB may work in engaging individuals to adhere to their medications.

The TPB is used to predict and explain behavior. Attitudes, subjective and social norms, and perceived behavioral control are components of behavioral intention. This theory suggests that utilizing a specific goal is helpful in constructing a change in behavior. For example, instead of utilizing a general goal of simply adhering to a medication regime, TPB would suggest stating a specific goal, such as by the end of the next month, the individual adhere to one primary medication regime. The creation of a specific goal (or goal intention), particularly in health promotion, has been linked to "implementation intention." While goal intentions provide a general goal (e.g., I want to lose weight), the implementation intention specifies the when, where, and how of the desired goal response (e.g., I will lose 20 pounds in 4 months; Brandstätter, Lengfelder, & Gollwitzer, 2001). Implementation intention is a self-regulatory strategy that helps alleviate the problems when striving for a particular goal. This means that goals that are furnished with implementation intentions are more easily attained. Orbell, Hodgkins, and Sheeran (1997) found that women who had made a strong goal intention to perform a breast exam in the next month were twice as likely to actually perform a breast examination compared to those without such an intention. Similarly, Sheeran and Orbell (1999) found that regular intake of vitamins were facilitated by implementation intentions. This research showcases that the use of specific goals, driven through implementation intentions, are far more successful in behavioral change.

"Behavioral intention" is defined as the likelihood that a person will engage in a specific behavior (Ajzen, 2002, 2011, 2012). Research has shown that behavioral intention is the best predictor of health behavior, such that those with positive behavioral intentions (e.g., to adhere to medication regimens) have better health and those with negative behavioral intentions (e.g., to avoid exercising) have poorer health (Ajzen, 2002, 2011; Taylor, 2010). This differs from implementation intention in that behavioral intention is more motivational while implementation intention is more volitional (Rise, Thompson, & Verplanken, 2003).

The other three primary components are structured as the predictors of behavioral intention. *Attitudes* regarding a health behavior include personal beliefs and valuations concerning the likely outcomes. For example, an older adult with a positive attitude toward medication is more likely to ascribe to the behavioral intention of adhering to the medication regime. *Subjective norms* refer to perceptions an individual holds regarding society's expectations of what they should be doing as well as motivation to comply with others' held beliefs. For example, if the subjective norm in a person's social group is to adhere to their medication regime, they are more likely to ascribe to the behavioral intention of adhering to the medication regime.

Finally, *perceived behavioral control* is considered to be how much control individuals believe they have to enact various behaviors and this typically transpires when people feel able to perform the action *and* when that action is perceived to lead to an expected outcome (Ajzen, 2002, 2011; Taylor, 2010). For example, an individual may believe that he or she can adhere successfully to the medication regime (perhaps due to increased health literacy), and thus is more likely to ascribe to the behavioral intention of adhering to the medication regime. Control, or perceived control, has shown positive effects in a multitude of studies (Ajzen, 2002, 2011; Rodin & Langer, 1977; Taylor, 2010), and is one of the stronger predictors in the TPB model. Rodin and Langer (1977) instituted an intervention in a nursing home to increase feelings of choice and personal responsibility. Across time, the results demonstrated that those receiving the intervention had lower mortality rates, were taking fewer medications, and overall, were happier, healthier, and more active.

Combining these factors has been useful in producing intentions regarding health behaviors leading to health behavior changes. It is important that people have both the ability and the motivation to obtain information relating to their health. Using these principles, the hydration project (described in the following) was conceived and implemented.

APPLICATIONS OF THEORETICAL MODELS TO HEALTHY LIVING

The previous sections focused on the building blocks for successful interventions, while the current section focuses on applications of said building blocks. In application, interventions (or the building of programs) begin with a *needs assessment*. A needs assessment identifies the "who, what, where, and why" of the need for a specific program (Stoecker, 2005).

Assessing the Need for Interventions

A quick search of the statistics on emergency room (ER) visits for adults over the age of 65 years revealed that there were 208,000 visits to the ER, logging dehydration as one of the primary diagnoses, and nearly 40 million visits where dehydration was the secondary diagnosis. If the average ER visit costs approximately $1,006 per day (Medicare), with an average stay of 6.5 days, that totals $1.36 billion dollars a year (Center for Disease Control and Prevention, 2007; Weinberg & Minaker, 1995). This section discusses the effects of dehydration and nutritional deficiencies, and then explores current and proposed intervention strategies.

You Can Lead a Horse to Water: The Effects of Dehydration

"Dehydration" is defined as the depletion in the total body water content of an individual (Benelam & Wyness, 2010). Dehydration can be caused by several factors, including disease, decreases in water intake, or a combination of both (Mentes, 2008). Hoffman (1991) suggests that adequate hydration in the older adult population is oftentimes a concern expressed by health care professionals, and yet is commonly overlooked in practice. One study reported that 48% of elders who were admitted into a hospital were diagnosed with having "chronic dehydration" (a fluid imbalance of longer duration usually caused by insufficient fluid intake; Bennett, Thomas, & Riegel, 2004). Further, it has been suggested by several researchers that dehydration is one of the most insidious and pressing problems in older adult populations (Himmelstein, Jones, & Woolhandler, 1983; Hoffman, 1991; Lavizzo-Mourney, 1987; Lavizzo-Mourney, Johnson, & Stolley, 1988). The "fix" of this problem seems relatively simple: dehydration can be easily avoided by consuming enough water; however, for the older adult population, several factors interfere with doing so.

Contributing factors pertaining to dehydration in older age include a reduced sense of thirst (Benelam & Wyness, 2010; Kenney & Chiu, 2001; Shimizu et al., 2012), prescription medications can interfere with how liquids taste (Benelam & Wyness, 2010; Feliciano et al., 2010; Graham, Suggs, & Sattely-Miller, 1998; Sansevero, 1997; Schiffman, 1997), peer gatherings increase the consumption of dehydrating beverages (i.e., coffee, alcohol), and a concern that drinking more fluids will result in incontinence (Feliciano et al., 2010). It is important to address the issue regarding dehydration within the elder population, specifically because elders who are dehydrated are at an increased risk for falls, urinary tract infections, and confusion; all of which could lead to ER visits and repeated hospitalizations (Campbell, 2011; Mentes, 2008). Hospitalization increases the health care costs for those individuals and provides a potentially traumatic experience for the elders (i.e., to be taken to the hospital for an emergency situation is fear inducing). Dehydration has also been linked to increased mortality rates in hospitalized older adults (Benelam & Wyness, 2010; Warren et al., 1994); as indicated earlier, in one sample, almost half of the elders admitted into hospital were dehydrated.

Taking into account all of these causes for dehydration in older adults and the detrimental outcomes of dehydration, it is imperative that interventions, specifically those geared toward increasing health literacy, are implemented and educational sessions about dehydration and its effects be held with this population. Feliciano and colleagues (2010) assessed barriers to hydration and developed nonintrusive interventions based on interviews with the participants. They found that providing consistent verbal and physical prompts and increasing the choice ("perceived behavioral control") of beverages can help increase individuals' fluid intake and decrease refusals of offered beverages (Feliciano et al., 2010). The information obtained in this study provides important preliminary data that suggests that the approaches taken are effective at overcoming some barriers that are associated with hydration in elders.

An Apple a Day: Nutritional Deficiencies

In addition to dehydration, nutritional deficiencies are another major health concern associated with the elders. "Nutritional deficiency" is defined as insufficient and/or inadequate nutritional intake. Nutritional deficiencies are harmful for all people, but elders in particular. Several reasons for this include increased difficultly in eating foods (e.g., dysphagia), and increase in food selectivity (i.e., food "pickiness") (Maitre et al., 2014).

Loss of appetite in those over 65 years of age, termed "anorexia of aging," is also a growing concern for this population. Anorexia of aging refers to the changes in the regulation of appetite and the lack of hunger associated with aging (Malafarina, Uriz-Otano, Gil-Guerrero, & Iniesta, 2013). When body weight declines, there is loss of both fat and muscle. This is a concern because weight loss in elders is associated with frailty, functional impairment, immune disorders, increased frequency of falls, low quality of life, and increased mortality (Johnson & Fischer, 2004; Thomas & Smith, 2009).

Reasons why elders might unintentionally lose weight include changes in routine (e.g., not being able to attend usual gatherings due to an injury), declining health (e.g., having increased risk for diabetes), environment (e.g., change in living circumstances), and declining social connections. Evidence has been found to support the notion that changes in environment, routine, and family/friend situations (i.e., loss of family members or other important persons) also negatively affect eating habits (Baker, 2007). Additional causes may include more internalized factors such as depression, feelings of loneliness, and cognitive losses, all which have been found to be associated with poor appetite and weight loss (Johnson & Fischer, 2004; Chan, Chan, Mok, & Tse, 2009).

Application: The Hydration Study

A small-scale, community-based program entitled "The Hydration Project" was designed to bring information to elders to educate them about the social and behavioral changes that aid in proper hydration utilizing the Theory of Planned Behavior (TPB). Community centers and living facilities of older adults (55+ years) were recruited. Pre- and posttest materials were constructed to assess the primary components of the TPB (i.e., attitudes, subjective norms, and perceived behavioral control). Further, both a behavioral (i.e., taste test of caffeinated vs. decaf teas) and educational (alternative hydrating options, how to recognize signs of dehydration, effects of dehydration, etc.) intervention was constructed for a 2-hour session.

The construction of the project was to provide individuals with detailed actions they could take to increase their health by utilizing goal intention (to drink more water) and implementation intention (i.e., providing water bottles, drink diaries, specific time period of increase). The participants ($N = 27$) ranged in age from 63 to 91 (74% Female), with $M = 77.37$ years ($SD = 7.14$). One of the primary foci was to help participants create goals and provide the steps toward goals in their hydration in the posttest assessment. In the posttest assessment, 100% felt they knew how to change their hydrating behaviors, 96% felt confident about drinking more hydrating liquids, 96% felt the steps were clear to the behavioral change, and 81% were planning to have a conversation about hydration with their friends. Further, in a 4-week follow-up with a daily hydration diary, 83% found the daily hydration diary to be a helpful tool in reminding them to reach their daily *Food and Drug Administration* (FDA) recommendations.[1]

The preliminary results reported here suggest that providing multiple types of behavioral and educational examples were helpful in providing participants with the tools necessary to be successful in implementing a plan to increase healthy hydration.

Application: Nostalgic Music and Daily Caloric Intake

Think about the introductory story, something as simple as music facilitating feelings of relaxation (physical and mental; Koch et al., 1998), and inducing pleasant and positive feelings (Blood & Zatorre, 2001; Menon & Levitin, 2005). For example, Sung, Chang, and Lee (2010) found that music therapy reduced levels of anxiety in older adults with dementia. They had two conditions wherein older adults either listened to music (intervention group) or went about their day as usual (control group). Elders in the music group received 30 minutes of music twice a week for 6 weeks during the midafternoon. Elders in the control group did not hear any music during the midafternoons. Their results indicated that elders in the intervention group had significantly lower anxiety from pretest to posttest.

Although it is important to reduce anxiety in elders during mealtime, likely leading to an increase in their consumption, there was a lack of empirical evidence to support this claim. Therefore, a recent study by two of the authors sought to fill this gap. Their study demonstrated that playing nostalgic music during mealtime for elder individuals increased food and drink consumption (Skaar & Kleyman, 2014). In this study, participants were randomly assigned to one of three different conditions during mealtimes (no music, classical music, or big band music). These music choices were selected because they were thought to be nostalgic for the elders. Results indicated that participants consumed more fluids and

---

1   This study is still in data collection, thus these are the preliminary results from two locations. For more information, e-mail the author.

calories during the morning meal, regardless of the music condition, but more at later meals with the presence of music (specifically big band). These findings have implications regarding time of day when simple stimuli could produce larger effects in the consumption of food or fluids. In the qualitative analyses, the morning meal was also the time of day when participants spent more time at the table, and engaged more with other residents. Further, the presence of music while dining, specifically big band (nostalgia) type music as an intervention, had a positive influence on increasing food and fluid consumption in elders (Skaar & Kleyman, 2014). Music-evoked nostalgia has been associated with feelings of being valued and the associated sense that life is meaningful (Routledge et al., 2011, Studies 1 & 2). Listening to nostalgic music with one's peers could foster feelings of well-being and a sense of shared history creating a sense of belonging. These feelings could result in longer time spent at the dinner table with more food and fluids being consumed.

Something as simple as playing nostalgia music during meal times could add to the quality of daily life for many elders and does not place demands on an aging body (Cohen, Bailey, & Nilsson, 2002). Weight loss and dehydration have been strong predictors of poor physical health in this population, and finding noninvasive ways to educate both patients and providers in ways to increase positive health behaviors is important as the large group of baby boomers approaches elder status. Overall, adding bits of nostalgia in elders' environments may increase overall health and well-being.

SUGGESTIONS FOR INTERVENTIONS TOWARD HEALTHY LIVING

Health care providers are increasingly utilizing technology to promote health awareness and provide health care programs (e.g., nutritional information, smoking cessation). Due to the increase of this medium to promote health information, it is not surprising that many of the initiatives to increase health literacy in older adults focus on computer literacy (increasing older adults' ability to find information on the Internet; Manafo & Wong, 2012). Although many older adults are willing to decrease their reliance on health care providers by seeking information on the Internet (Manafo & Wong, 2012), many older adults are not comfortable using the Internet and may have difficulty or low to no interest in seeking information in this way (Cresci & Novak, 2012). Patients in the latter categories would prefer to turn to their health care professionals for this information.

Older adults have unique challenges with obtaining and retaining information regarding their health that might include cognitive limitations such as Alzheimer's (Kaphingst, Goodman, MacMillan, Carpenter, & Griffey, 2014) or physical limitations such as hearing loss. Therefore, it is important to implement interventions that are easy to adapt to a variety of situations and to the individuals receiving the information (Frosch & Elwyn, 2014).

Simple Solutions of Health Literacy Through the Environment

As outlined, we believe it is critical for elders to be given the necessary tools and education in order to increase their health literacy skills. There are, however, other low-cost intervention strategies that can be implemented to assist the elder population beyond health literacy. As mentioned, individuals' moods and emotional states can impact their food and water consumption (Blood & Zatorre, 2001; Menon & Levitin, 2005), which can lead to negative health impacts. By uplifting individuals' emotions or moods, however, we might be able to increase food and water consumption. Specifically, environmental factors, such as noise (Garre-Olmo et al., 2012), lighting (Küller, Ballal, Laike, Mikellides, & Tonello, 2006), and wall color can impact people's moods (Sobal & Wansink, 2007). Making small changes in elders' environments may assist in increasing elders' consumption of food and fluids in creative, low cost, and innovative ways. Chen, Hsu, Tung, and Pan (2013) indicated that a path to health literacy could be forged through health education, health management, and disease knowledge, which may indirectly promote healthier lifestyles.

CONCLUSION

Interventions that are created to help patients achieve improved health outcomes and receive care consistent with their personal preferences might lead to lower medical costs and increase patient satisfaction (Frosch & Elwyn, 2014). Technology is being used as a conduit for health information; it is imperative that health professionals understand that elders may not be aware that this information is available, and even if they are aware, elders might not have the ability or the means to access this information (Cresci & Novak, 2012). It is important to find ways to create and implement low-cost interventions that increase health behavior, such as small changes in elders' environment and applied educational programing. This information should be easy to understand and implement. If interventions are to be successful, health care providers must have the ability and motivation to communicate this information as well as the ability to put effective changes in place. Patients must also have the capacity to process this information (Kaphingst et al., 2014) as well as the motivation to change behaviors and longtime habits.

The primary point of this chapter was to highlight some of the pitfalls regarding the health care system as they relate to older adults. Specifically, interventions to increase health literacy need to become more readily available to elders. Today, it seems that health care providers are tasked with more responsibilities and patients than they can care for. Due to time restraints and workloads placed upon them, it is near impossible to provide all patients with the information required for them to either be fully informed about their health care or to know how and where to acquire this information. We outlined several areas in which elder individuals' health may be negatively impacted due to dehydration and nutritional deficiencies. We suggested that by increasing health literacy and by providing environmental, educational, and behavioral interventions with this aging population, we may be able to reduce problems caused by dehydration and malnourishment.

REFERENCES

Ajzen, I. (2002). Residual effects of past on later behavior: Habituation and reasoned action perspectives. *Personality and Social Psychology Review, 6*, 107–122.

Ajzen, I. (2011). The theory of planned behaviour: Reactions and reflections. *Psychology and Health, 26*, 1113–1127.

Ajzen, I. (2012). The theory of planned behavior. In P. M. Van Lange, A. W. Kruglanski, & E. T. Higgins (Eds.), *Handbook of theories of social psychology* (Vol. 1, pp. 438–459). Thousand Oaks, CA: Sage.

Baker, H. (2007). Nutrition in the elderly: An overview. *Geriatrics, 62*(7), 28–34.

Benelam, B., & Wyness, L. (2010). Hydration and health: A review. *Nutrition Bulletin, 35*(1), 3–25.

Bennett, J. A., Thomas, V., & Riegel, B. (2004). Unrecognized chronic dehydration in older adults: Examining prevalence rate and risk factors. *Journal of Gerontological Nursing, 30*, 22–28.

Blood, A. J., & Zatorre, R. J. (2001). Intensely pleasurable responses to music correlate with activity in brain regions implicated in reward and emotion. *Proceedings of the National Academy of Sciences, 98*, 11818–11823.

Brandstätter, V., Lengfelder, A., & Gollwitzer, P. M. (2001). Implementation intentions and efficient action initiation. *Journal of Personality and Social Psychology, 81*(5), 946–960.

Campbell, N. (2011). Dehydration: Why is it still a problem? *Nursing Times, 107*, 12–15.

Centers for Disease Control and Prevention. (2007). *National hospital discharge survey* [Data file]. Retrieved from http://www.cdc.gov/nchs/nhds/nhds_products.htm

Centers for Disease Control and Prevention. (2014). *National diabetes statistics report (2014)*. Atlanta, Georgia, U.S. Department of Health and Human Services, Centers for Disease Control and Prevention.

Chan, M., Chan, E., Mok, E., & Kwan Tse, F. (2009). Effect of music on depression levels and physiological responses in community-based older adults. *International Journal of Mental Health Nursing, 18*, 285–294.

Chen, J., Hsu, H., Tung, H., & Pan, L. (2013). Effects of health literacy to self-efficacy and preventive care utilization among older adults. *Geriatrics & Gerontology International, 13*, 70–76.

Chen, P. (2013). For new doctors, 8 minutes per patient. *The New York Times*. Retrieved from http://well.blogs.nytimes.com/2013/05/30/for-new-doctors-8-minutes-per-patient/?_r=0

Cohen, A., Bailey, B., & Nilsson, T. (2002). The importance of music to seniors. *Psychomusicology, 18*, 89–102.

Cresci, M. K., & Novak, J. M. (2012). Information technologies as health management tools: Urban elders' interest and ability in using the Internet. *Educational Gerontology, 38*, 491–506.

Dugdale, D. C., Epstein, R., & Pantilat, S. Z. (1999). Time and the patient–physician relationship. *Journal of General Internal Medicine, 14*, S34–S40.

Feliciano, L., LeBlanc, L. A., & Feeney, B. J. (2010). Assessment and management of barriers to fluid intake in community dwelling older adults. *Journal of Behavioral Health and Medicine, 1*, 3–14.

Frosch, D. L., & Elwyn, G. (2014). Don't blame patients, engage them: Transforming health systems to address health literacy. *Journal of Health Communication, 19*, 10–14.

Garre-Olmo, J., López-Pousa, S., Turon-Estrada, A., Juvinyà, D., Ballester, D., & Vilalta-Franch, J. (2012). Environmental determinants of quality of life in nursing home residents with severe dementia. *Journal of the American Geriatrics Society, 60*, 1230–1236.

Harris-Kojetin L., Sengupta M., Park-Lee E., & Valverde R. (2013) *Long-term care services in the United States: 2013 overview*. National Center for Health Statistics. Vital and Health Statistics, 3, vi–55.

Himmelstein, D. U., Jones, A. A., & Woolhandler, S. (1983). Hypernatremic dehydration in nursing home patients: An indicator of neglect. *Journal of the American Geriatrics Society, 31*, 466–471.

Hoffman, N. B. (1991). Dehydration in the elderly: Insidious and manageable. *Geriatrics, 46*, 35–38.

Hofstede, G. (1980). *Culture's consequences: International differences in work-related values*. Beverly Hills, CA: Sage.

Ishikawa, H., & Yano, E. (2008). Patient health literacy and participation in the healthcare process. *Health Expectations, 11*, 113–122.

Johnson, M., & Fischer, J. G. (2004). Eating and appetite: Common problems and practical remedies. *Generations, 28*, 11–17.

Kaphingst, K. A., Goodman, M. S., MacMillan, W. D., Carpenter, C. R., & Griffey, R. T. (2014). Effect of cognitive dysfunction on the relationship between age and health literacy. *Patient Education and Counseling, 95*, 218–225.

Kenney, W. L., & Chiu, P. (2001). Influence of age on thirst and fluid intake. *Medical Science Sports and Exercise, 33*, 1524–1532.

Koch, Kain, Ayoub, & Rosenbaum (1998). The sedative and analgesic sparing effect of music. *Anesthesiology, 89*, 300–306.

Küller, R., Ballal, S., Laike, T., Mikellides, B., & Tonello, G. (2006). The impact of light and colour on psychological mood: A cross-cultural study of indoor work environments. *Ergonomics, 49*, 1496–1507.

Kutner, M., Greenburg, E., Jin, Y., & Paulsen, C. (2006). *The health literacy of America's adults: Results from the 2003 national assessment of adult literacy.* NCES 2006-483 (pp. 1–60). Washington, DC: National Center for Education Statistics.

Lavizzo-Mourney, R. J. (1987). Dehydration in the elderly: A short review. *Journal of the National Medical Association, 79*, 1033–1038.

Lavizzo-Mourney, R. J., Johnson, J., & Stolly, P. (1988). Risk factors for dehydration among elderly nursing home residents. *Journal of the American Geriatrics Society, 36*, 213–218.

Maitre, I., Van Wymelbeke, V., Amand, M., Vigneau, E., Issanchou, S., & Sulmont-Rossé, C. (2014). Food pickiness in the elderly: Relationship with dependency and malnutrition. *Food Quality and Preference, 32*(Part B), 145–151.

Malafarina, V., Uriz-Otano, F., Gil-Guerrero, L., & Iniesta, R. (2013). The anorexia of ageing: Physiopathology, prevalence, associated comorbidity and mortality. A systematic review. *Maturitas, 74*, 293–302.

Manafo, E., & Wong, S. (2012). Health literacy programs for older adults: A systematic literature review. *Health Education Research, 27*, 947–960.

Menon, V., & Levitin, D. J. (2005). The rewards of music listening: Response and physiological connectivity of the mesolimbic system. *Neuroimage, 28*, 175–184.

Mentes, J. C. (2008). Managing oral hydration. In E. Capezuti, D. Zwicker, M. Mezey, T. T. Fulmer, D. Gray-Miceli, & M. Kluger (Eds.), *Evidence-based geriatric nursing protocols for best practice* (3rd ed., pp. 369–390). New York, NY: Springer Publishing Company.

Moody, H. R., & Sasser, J. R. (2015). *Concepts and controversies* (8th ed., pp. 269–300). London, UK: Sage.

Orbell, S., Hodgkins, S., & Sheeran, P. (1997). Implementation intentions and the theory of planned behavior. *Personality and Social Psychology Bulletin, 23*, 945–954.

Rabin, R. (2014). *15-minute visits take a toll on the doctor–patient relationship.* Retrieved from www.medscape.com/viewarticle/823992

Ratzan, S. C., & Parker, R. M. (2006). Health literacy: Identification and response. *Journal of Health Communication: International Perspectives, 11*, 713–715.

Ribbe, M. W., Ljunggren, G., Steel, K., Topinkova, E., Hawes, C., Ikegami, Henrad, J. C., & Jonnson, V. (1997). Nursing homes in 10 nations: A comparison between countries and settings. *Age and Ageing, 26*, 3–12.

Rise, J., Thompson, M., & Verplanken, B. (2003). Measuring implementation intentions in the context of the theory of planned behavior. *Scandinavian Journal of Psychology, 44*, 87–95.

Rodin, J., & Langer, E. J. (1977). Long-term effects of a control-relevant intervention with the institutionalized aged. *Journal of Personality and Social Psychology, 35,* 897–902.

Rosenthal, R., & Jacobson, L. (1968). Pygmalion in the classroom. *The Urban Review, 3,* 16–20.

Ross, L., Greene, D., & House, P. (1977). The false consensus effect: An egocentric bias in social perception and attribution processes. *Journal of Experimental Social Psychology, 13*(3), 279–301.

Rossato-Bennett, M. (Producer/Director). (2014). *Alive Inside* [Motion Picture]. United States: MVD Entertainment.

Routledge, C., Arndt, J., Wildschut, T., Sedikides, C., Hart, C. M., Juhl, J., & Schlotz, W. (2011). The past makes the present meaningful: Nostalgia as an existential resource. *Journal of Personality and Social Psychology, 101,* 638–652.

Rudd, R. E. (2007). Health literacy skills of U.S. adults. *American Journal of Health Behavior, 31*(Suppl. 1), S8–S18.

Sansevero, A. C. (1997). Dehydration in the elderly: Strategies for prevention and management. *The Nurse Practitioner, 22,* 41–42, 51–57, 63–66.

Schiffman, S., Graham, B., Suggs, M., & Sattely-Miller, E. (1998). Effect of psychotropic drugs on taste responses in young and elderly persons. (pp. 732–737). New York: New York Acad Sciences.

Schillinger, D., Grumbach, K., Piette, J., Wang, F., Osmond, D., Daher, C., & Bindman, A. B. (2002). Association of health literacy with diabetes outcomes. *Journal of the American Medical Association, 288,* 475–482.

Sheeran, P., & Orbell, S. (1999). Implementation intentions and repeated behaviors: Augmenting the predictive validity of the theory of planned behavior. *European Journal of Social Psychology, 29,* 349–370.

Shimizu, M., Kinoshita, K., Hattori, K., Ota, Y., Kanai, T., Kobayashi, H., & Tokuda, Y. (2012). Physical signs of dehydration in the elderly. *Internal Medicine, 51*(10), 1207–1210.

Skaar, T. B., & Kleyman, K. S. (2014, February). *Sounds delicious: The effects of nostalgic music on increased food consumption in older adults.* Poster session presented at the annual meeting of the Society for Personality and Social Psychology (SPSP), Austin, TX.

Sobal, J., & Wansink, B. (2007). Kitchenscapes, tablescapes, platescapes, and foodscapes: Influences of microscale built environments on food intake. *Environment and Behavior, 39,* 124–142.

Spangler, P. F., Risley, T. R., & Bilyew, D. D. (1984). The management of dehydration and incontinence in nonambulatory geriatric patients. *Journal of Applied Behavior Analysis, 17,* 397–401.

Spencer, L. M., Schooley, M. W., Anderson, L. A., Kochtitzky, C. S., DeGroff, A. S., Devlin, H. M., & Mercer, S. L. (2013). Seeking best practices: A conceptual framework for planning and improving evidence-based practices. *Preventing Chronic Disease: Public Health Research, Practice, and Policy, 10,* 130–186.

Stoecker, R. (2005). Is community informatics good for communities? Questions confronting an emerging field. *Journal of Community Informatics, 3,* 13–26.

Sung, H., Chang, A. M., & Lee, W. (2010). A preferred music listening intervention to reduce anxiety in older adults with dementia in nursing homes. *Journal of Clinical Nursing, 19*, 1056–1064.

Taylor, S. E. (2010). Health. In S. Fiske, D. Gilbert, & G. Lindzey (Eds.), *Handbook of social psychology* (5th ed., Vol. 1, pp. 698–723). Hoboken, NJ: Wiley.

Thomas, D., & Smith, M. (2009). The effect of music on caloric consumption among nursing home residents with dementia of the Alzheimer's type. *Activities, Adaptation & Aging, 33*, 1–16.

U.S. Department of Health and Human Services (HRSA). (2014). *Shortage designation: Health professional shortage areas & medically underserved areas/populations.* Retrieved from http://www.hrsa.gov/shortage

Warren, J. L., Bacon, W. E., Harris, T., McBean, A. M., Foley, D., & Phillips, C. (1994). The burden and outcomes associated with dehydration among U.S. elderly, 1991. *American Journal of Public Health, 84*, 1265–1269.

Weinberg, A. D., & Minaker, K. L. (1995). Dehydration: Evaluation and management in older adults. Council on Scientific Affairs, American Medical Association. *Journal of the American Medical Association, 274*, 1552–1556.

Weiss, L. J., & Blustein, J. (1996). Faithful patients: The effect of long-term physician–patient relationships on the costs and use of health care by older Americans. *American Journal of Public Health, 86*, 1742–1747. doi: 10.2105/AJPH.86.12.1742

Welton, J. (2007). *Mandatory hospital nurse to patient staffing ratios: Time to take a different approach.* Retrieved from http://www.nursingworld.org/MainMenuCategories/ANAMarketplace/ANAPeriodicals/OJIN/TableofContents/Volume122007/No3Sept07/MandatoryNursetoPatientRatios.htm

World Health Organization (WHO). (1998). Division of health promotion, education and communications health education and health promotion unit. *Health promotion glossary.* World Health Organization, Geneva. Retrieved from http://www.who.int/healthpromotion/conferences/7gchp/track2/en

CHAPTER 12

Cultural Competence and Health Literacy

IRIS FEINBERG, DAPHNE GREENBERG, AND AMANI TALWAR

A broad and overarching goal of health care delivery, health promotion, and health education is to improve the health and quality of life for all groups of people across all cultures and all life stages (Centers for Disease Control and Prevention [CDC], 2015a). In 2008, more than 33% of the U.S. population identified as belonging to a racial or ethnic minority population, 51% of the U.S. population were women, 23% of the population lived in rural areas, and 20% spoke a language other than English at home (CDC, 2015a, 2015b; U.S. Census Bureau). Acknowledging cultural differences in health care and health education is important because culture forms one's perspectives on health, wellness, disease, and treatment, and these perspectives can be vastly different within individuals, groups, and populations. It is essential, therefore, for health care and health education providers to understand how culture and health are intertwined. This chapter will discuss the intersection of health literacy and culture as they relate to older adults.

HEALTH LITERACY

Health literacy is typically defined as the ability to obtain, read, understand, and use health care information to make meaningful health decisions and follow instructions for prevention and treatment (Kindig, Panzer, & Nielsen-Bohlman, 2004; Osborne, 2012; Parker et al., 1999; Speros, 2009). According to the National Association of Adult Literacy study in 2003, individuals aged 65 and older had the lowest health literacy scores of any age bracket (Kutner, Greenberg, Jin, & Paulsen, 2006). The number of older people in the United States is expected to double to 72 million people by 2030; additionally, by 2050, one in four older adults is projected to be from one of the four populations designated as minority: African American, Asian, Hispanic, and Other (U.S. Census Bureau). Thus, the United States will have a large older adult segment of the population that combines the highest demand for health care services of any age group, the lowest health literacy scores, and many who will belong to racial and ethnic minorities.

The move to patient-centered care and shared decision making as standards of care puts patients in the difficult position of needing to acquire disease knowledge and complex self-care skills through written and verbal instructions (Logan et al., 2015; Ownby, Waldrop-Valverde, & Taha, 2012; Speros, 2009). Older adults from marginalized groups who have low background health knowledge and low reading skills may be too uncomfortable to ask questions of their health provider (Findley, 2015; Speros, 2009). If information is not conveyed in a culturally and literacy-level appropriate way, it will not be understood or acted upon. A fundamental goal of health literacy for older adults is to improve their access to health information and help them use it effectively to make informed choices and exert greater control over their lives (Bennett, Chen, Soroui, & White, 2009; Findley, 2015; Fortier & Bishop, 2004; Kutob et al., 2013; Lyons, Dunson-Strane, & Sherman, 2014; Purdie & McCrindle, 2002; Ziegahn & Ton, 2011). This interactive health literacy happens when individuals acquire and apply both disease knowledge and practical knowledge in reading and numeracy as well as communicate well with health providers, learn how to solve problems, and make meaningful health-related decisions (Aguilera, Dailey, & Perez, 2008; Manafo & Wong, 2012; Osborne, 2012; Rubin, 2014; Zamora & Clingerman, 2011).

CULTURAL COMPETENCY AND HEALTH LITERACY

Culturally competent health literacy for older adults integrates issues related to aging with language differences, cultural differences, and an awareness of differences in health beliefs and behaviors. Common elements that individuals use to form their cultural identities include language, customs, beliefs, values, actions, and institutions. Often specific to racial, ethnic, socioeconomic, religious, social, peer, and/or geographic groups, culture influences the way people communicate and present themselves in all aspects of life (Betancourt, Green, Carrillo, & Ananeh-Firempong, 2003; Galambos, 2003; National Center for Cultural Competence [NCCC]). Internal to each culture are patterns and core values, and, as such, cultural boundaries are created organically

(Galambos, 2003; NCCC; Yeo, 2009). People also have their own cultural histories, biases, ideas, and values, which can create language barriers and cultural mismatches (Aguilera et al., 2008; Guy, 1999; Lie, Carter-Pokras, Braun, & Coleman, 2012; Office of Minority Health [OMH], U.S. Department of Health and Human Services; Yeo, 2009). Oftentimes, these cultural boundaries are not clear because each individual belongs to more than one cultural group, which causes the intersection and interaction of different cultural values within each of us. Cross-cultural communication, the ability to appropriately and effectively communicate across those boundaries, is a critical skill as there are few instances where people interact solely with others in their own culture (Langer, 2008; NCCC; Yeo, 2009).

Culture also plays a critical role in how individuals view health, health care, and health systems. Inherent in these views are the systems of beliefs that govern what causes illness and wellness, how the body works, how diseases are treated or cured, and who should participate in the delivery of health care and health-related services (Betancourt et al., 2003; Galambos, 2003; Koh, Garcia, & Alvarez, 2014; Lie et al., 2012; Whaley, 2000). For example, many groups within Western indus-trialized societies see disease as a result of natural scientific phenomena, while many groups within Eastern societies believe that illness is the result of the supernatural (Aguilera et al., 2008; Langer, 2008; Whaley, 2000; Yeo, 2009). Cultural beliefs play a role in how patient education is perceived, what kinds of compliance measures are likely to be adhered to, and why health promotion interventions may work for some but not for others (Aguilera et al., 2008; Betancourt et al., 2003; Langer, 2008; NCCC; Yeo, 2009). For example, military veterans, who are part of a cul-ture that emphasizes discipline and hierarchy, may have a very difficult time questioning authority, even if those questions are simply to access more information (Hsu, 2010). In order to cross these and other linguis-tic and cultural boundaries, health care and health education providers must develop cultural competence, which is the ability to relate to and interact with people of different cultures in a respectful and responsive manner.

There are many challenges inherent in providing literacy-level appropriate health education while also considering culturally distin-guishing features. For instance, a culturally distinguishing feature is peer affiliation, which can influence one's cultural norms. For example, studies of military veterans show an organizational culture replete with certain behavioral norms and expectations, which can create difficulty integrating civilian and military identities (Koenig, Maguen, Monroy,

Mayott, & Seal, 2014). In particular, there is a norm of organization, rules, and performing behaviors without question (Koenig et al., 2014). As another example, African American culture values strong kinship bonds, informal support networks (family, church, and community), and a strong sense of self-sufficiency and pride (Whaley, 2000). Other strong cultural values are a heightened sense of religious belief relating to illness (God as healer) that may cause a delay in seeking treatment or taking individual control over health behaviors (Levin, Chatters, & Taylor, 2005; Whaley, 2000). Geography can also play a role in how health education is delivered and received; rural citizens may have greater access to community-level care than to medical clinics and hospitals due to a wider geographic distribution of health providers. Their health problems may be more serious by the time they are diagnosed or by the time they are treated (Bolin & Bellamy, 2011; Meit, 2004) since their access to health care may be restricted due to distance.

Latino culture values "respeto" (respect), "la familia" (family), and "personalismo" (trust of others by developing personal relationships) (Whaley, 2000). These values directly inform how health messages are received as they guide such behaviors as being deferential toward others, which may lead to not getting clarification, expecting family members to provide explanations and support. Belief in these values may also lead to a lack of trust in health providers who speak directly and do not develop a personal relationship with a patient (Keller et al., 2012; Whaley, 2000). Many Asian cultures hold beliefs such as a collectivist orientation (group needs are greater than individual needs), an indirect communication style (expecting others to understand what is meant instead of what is directly said), face maintenance (not wanting to impose on others), and shame orientation (a concern about behaviors that bring embarrassment), all of which are very different than Western behaviors (Whaley, 2000).

Finally, there are linguistic challenges to consider. For example, Spanish speakers may understand and use the English language, but there may be different meanings and connotations in even everyday words. One simple example is the word "once" which English speakers know to mean one time. Spanish speakers may read "once" as "on-say" in Spanish, which means the number 11; this could drastically change the number of pills one takes or the number of times one does something. Another linguistic challenge is the common use in English of negatives, for example, "You don't want to be sick, do you?" which may be difficult for non-native English speakers to translate and comprehend.

CULTURE, HEALTH LITERACY, AND INTERVENTIONS

A perusal of the literature points to very few examples of health literacy intervention studies on older adults with a focus on cultural differences. We highlight a few examples that we feel depict how culture is important to consider when designing health literacy interventions. The selected studies represent a variety of different cultural aspects— language, ethnicity, and geography. Although these studies were not focused primarily on cultural competency, we highlight cultural awareness issues that are reflected in each study.

Valle, Yamada, and Matiella (2006) examined the health education impact of a fotonovela (photo novel) about Alzheimer's disease with 111 older Spanish-speaking adults. The fotonovela was delivered by a facilitator in a guided educational session and then left with the participants. Prior knowledge of and experience with dementia and Alzheimer's disease was measured both pre- and post-intervention; results showed a significant increase in knowledge on five out of the six study questions. Researchers also evaluated whether the participants liked the fotonovela, found it informative, and/or found it understandable. Results indicated that the young older group of participants (age range 55–64), and women in all age cohorts (55–64, 65–74, 75 plus) found the fotonovela more informative than others. A high rate of study participants (41%) also shared the fotonovela with others who were not part of the study.

This study shows that providing health information in an individual's first language and in a format that is culturally sensitive and meaningful can increase individual health knowledge (Guy, 1999; Koh et al., 2014; Langer, 2008; Orem, 2005; Osborne, 2012; Whaley, 2000; Yeo, 2009). The Latino culture values using education entertainment as a way to combine factual and emotional information that can assist in decision making (Castaneda, Organista, Rodriguez, & Check, 2013; Tufte, 2009; Valle et al., 2006). The delivery modality of health education materials—for example, using a fotonovela format for a Hispanic audience—increases the likelihood that an individual will be able to retain the information presented (Castaneda et al., 2013; Tufte, 2009; Valle et al., 2006). Popular culture fotonovelas are often recirculated through the Hispanic community; this educational fotonovela was also shared, indicating a common cultural phenomenon (Flora, 1980; Valle et al., 2006).

In a study by Fitzpatrick and colleagues (2012), older Asian adults provided their perspectives on cardiovascular health through the use of photovoice, a qualitative methodology using photographs taken by participants. The participants were Chinese, Vietnamese, and Korean older adults, with mean age 71.6 years ($n = 23$). Bilingual facilitators were trained in the photovoice methodology (one in Cantonese, one in Vietnamese, and one in Korean), and all written materials were translated into these languages as well. The facilitators explained the photovoice methodology to participants, including how to use the camera and take good pictures. At the second session, participants presented their photographs; facilitators led the group discussion based on themes of what heart health is, what helps and hurts your heart, and barriers to care and education. This study brought out commonalities and differences in perspectives of heart disease held by different Asian groups. For example, all three groups were concerned with stress; however, while the Chinese and Vietnamese participants felt that stress was induced by external factors that cause fear or anxiety, a Korean perspective was that the internal factor of loneliness brought on stress.

This creative study methodology was acceptable to participants, and helped give voice to the beliefs, needs, and knowledge of these vulnerable Chinese, Vietnamese, and Korean older adults. Using visual images rather than direct language was a way to value the indirect communication style favored by Asians (Whaley, 2000), and gave voice to both ideas about health and a way to learn what these individuals knew about health and health care. Another highlight of the study was that care was taken to honor the three different groups within the Asian culture, each of which may have very different belief structures and knowledge about health and health care, rather than combining the three into one generalized group (Galambos, 2003; Koh et al., 2014; Langer, 2008).

A multiple intervention program called "Health Enhancement for Rural Elderly" was run with older rural adults in Montana by Young, Weinert, and Spring (2012). One intervention was the delivery of Health Information Webinars, which had 152 participants (no mean age provided). Health Information Webinars consisted of five monthly health information webinars broadcast to four rural communities. The intent of the webinars was to increase health literacy skills with a central theme of how to obtain, evaluate, and use web-based information. Senior community centers were provided with necessary equipment to host these webinars.

Education is often hard to deliver in rural areas because of the vast distances between people and communities; therefore, the use of computer technology to share and provide health information seems like a natural fit. In this study, the participants found the information useful and a majority indicated that they would recommend the webinars to others. The participants indicated that the Internet was a valuable source of health information; however, only about half of the participants had Internet access at home, which limits the usability and sustainability of a program like this (Butler et al., 2011). Therefore, being able to access the webinars in the community centers shows the importance of providing access to individuals in rural areas. Providing the webinars in a setting such as a community center or library helps develop this concept into a community-wide model where older adults, their families, and their caregivers could attend together, which may be important in sustaining and enhancing health education (Bolin & Bellamy, 2011; Butler et al., 2011; Horrell, Stephens, & Breheny, 2014; Meit, 2004).

FEDERAL POLICY INITIATIVES

There are various federal policy initiatives to enhance cultural competence in health care, including the 2010 National Action Plan to Improve Health Literacy. This plan focuses on decreasing barriers to health care access and improving informed decision making by encouraging the use of evidence-based health literacy research in all areas—including cultural competency—to inform change (Office of Disease Prevention and Health Promotion, 2010). The Plain Writing Act of 2010, another federal initiative, requires federal agencies to use plain language in any document that provides information about federal benefits or services, including health information (Plain Writing Act, 2010). Plain language helps individuals who have low literacy from different cultures understand health care messages in ways that may be more meaningful to them. The 2011 Health and Human Services Strategic Action Plan to reduce racial and ethnic health disparities includes updating and disseminating national standards on linguistically and culturally appropriate health care services (OMH). These standards, known as Culturally and Linguistically Appropriate Services (CLAS), are broken into three thematic sections and provide a framework within which health care providers can enhance their services to be the most responsive to cultural health beliefs and practices, preferred languages, health literacy levels, and other communication needs (OMH). The first section is Governance, Leadership, and Workforce and provides a blueprint for building culturally and linguistically health-literate organizations. The second section, Communication and Language Assistance, specifies standards for appropriate and timely health-related language assistance as well as easy-to-understand health organization signage and materials. The final section is Engagement, Continuous Improvement, and Accountability, and provides guidelines for quality improvement, evaluation, and community engagement in health organizations. While not mandated by law, the CLAS standards have been adopted by many organizations for consideration and implementation at the highest levels (board and governance) through day-to-day activities (language assistance, community engagement, and education) (Koh et al., 2014).

HEALTH CARE WORKERS

Since health care workers are the ones who deliver a majority of health information, it is essential that cultural and linguistic sensitivity is included in their training. Approximately 18,000 new doctors graduate every year from 134 accredited U.S. medical schools; all are trained in the science and art of practicing medicine and have learned how to make appropriate life or death decisions in situations that are often fraught with risk, high emotions, and chaos (Association of American Medical Colleges, 2011). Cultural sensitivity training is offered either as a stand-alone class or is integrated into existing lectures in many medical, nursing, and pharmaceutical schools (Flores, Gee, & Kastner, 2000; Koh et al., 2014). One of the most important components to providing effective health care is learning how to communicate with an increasingly varied cultural, ethnic, and linguistic population so that people get the care they deserve and need, regardless of background.

In addition to what may be offered as part of the medical school curriculum, many private and public organizations offer courses in cultural and linguistic sensitivity as part of Continuing Medical Education credits. Their goal is to enable physicians and other clinical staff to broaden attitudes and understanding about their diverse patient populations (Betancourt & Green, 2010; Betancourt, Green, & Carrillo, 2002) by increasing both knowledge about sociocultural diversity and hands-on skills. Organizations like the U.S. Department of Health and Human Services also offer health literacy and intercultural training and education for health care professionals including workshops, online training, guidance on creating a health literacy plan for medical organizations, and resources for material development (Center for Linguistic and Cultural Competence in Health Care [CLCCHC], Office of Minority Health, U.S. Department of Health and Human Services). There is also continued recognition and implementation of mandated and continuing education offerings in cultural sensitivity and health literacy training for pharmacists, nurses, physical therapists, and other health care providers (Betancourt & Green, 2010; Betancourt et al., 2002; Koh et al., 2014; CLCCHC, Office of Minority Health, U.S. Department of Health and Human Services).

SUMMARY

While the literature describes the great need for cultural competence in health care delivery and health education, we were able to identify very few health literacy research interventions that specifically study cultural issues for older adults. This is unfortunate because individuals define health and illness through the lens of their own cultural backgrounds, which is made even more complicated by the intersection of many different cultural affiliations. For example, a person could be female, Hispanic, 65, an immigrant, and live in a rural community, or a person could be a male African American military veteran from a Caribbean background. This interaction of cultures affects choice of health provider, description of symptoms, consideration of treatment options, and whether treatment will be adhered to (Andrulis & Brach, 2007), and it is difficult, if not impossible, to know which cultural position may have the strongest impact. While this chapter focuses on patients, culture also affects the health care provider, staff, institution, industry, and caregiver; health care providers and health care systems need interventions that can cut across cultural and linguistic boundaries. These population-specific differences are often responsible for not only poor health quality outcomes, but also for a lack of efficiency within the health care system; according to a study by the Joint Center for Political and Economic Studies, elimination of these social disparities would have reduced direct medical care expenditures by $229.4 billion between 2003 and 2006 (LaViest, Gaskin, & Richard, 2009). Creating culturally competent health care and health education delivery can increase quality of life outcomes, decrease health disparities, and act as a business strategy for the medical industry to increase their market share (Betancourt et al., 2002). In their 2002 field report, Betancourt, Green, and Carrillo discussed opportunities to develop three different types of cultural competence in the health care delivery system—organizational (within the health care workforce), systemic (within the systems of care like hospitals and clinics), and clinical (within the provider community). By reducing cultural dissonance and increasing cultural competence, differences in cultural experiences can be valued in the delivery of education, care and services.

CASE STUDY

Physicians in an urban neighborhood gerontology clinic were concerned that their "young" patients ages 65 to 74 were too sedentary, and decided to try an organized group-walking intervention. Two-thirds of the clinic patients were African American and the remaining were Asian American and Latino. The walking group would be led by one of the nurses in the clinic; walking would last 1 hour and would start at the clinic on Monday, Wednesday, and Friday mornings at 9 a.m. Patients who participated would get a pedometer and access to an online fitness program to keep track of their progress. On the first Monday, 10 African Americans, 4 Latinos, and 0 Asians showed up for the walk. The group walked to a nearby high school, walked around the track several times, had a water break, and then walked back to the clinic. They then spent 15 minutes logging on to the computer at the clinic and recording their results. On Wednesday, only three African Americans showed up for the walk. On Friday, 12 African Americans and six Latinos who had not participated on Monday showed up for the walk. On each day, new participants stayed after the walk to learn how to log on to the computer and record their results. The same thing happened the second week. The clinic staff was puzzled at the changing structure of the group, as well as at the absence of any of the Asian American patients. They decided to interview a selection of patients to see why they did or did not participate in the walking group.

Responses for participation were varied. The African Americans belonged to a neighborhood church prayer meeting that met every Wednesday morning; their primary affiliation was to their church where they had developed strong bonds and support. The group of Latinos who came on the first day did not feel comfortable in their English language or computer skills, so they did not come back. They also commented that they did not want to walk around the high school track because their grandchildren went to that school and the older adults didn't want to be seen by them. A group of Asian American patients were interviewed; the two reasons that were reported most often were face saving and shame (they were concerned that they could not walk for an hour and did not want to slow down the rest of the group). The physicians and nurses realized that they could easily customize the program—and their expectations for outcomes—for the different cultures represented in their practice by considering the values and beliefs of each racial/ethnic group. The staff made several changes to the program. A written journal was added for those who preferred to write in journals rather than use the computer-based online fitness program. Everyone was welcome to attend each walking session; however, Wednesday was customized for the Latino community with a different route and a bilingual walking leader. A separate Asian American group was invited on Thursday for a shorter walk with an Asian American physician's assistant. In this way, cultural values and norms for each race/ethnicity were honored and participation in the walking program increased.

DISCUSSION QUESTIONS

1. What are some significant areas of conflict that might impede culturally and literacy appropriate communication with patients and their health care providers?
2. Think of recent health communication materials you have seen. Describe their cultural and literacy appropriate content, messages, and graphics. Identify the target audience.
3. Suppose you had to take your elderly parent or grandparent to the hospital emergency room in another country where the majority culture of the country was very different from your grandparent's culture. What types of things would you need to consider in order to make sure that you and your parent/grandparent got the best possible care?

REFERENCES

Aguilera, C., Dailey, W. H., & Perez, M. A. (2008). Aging and health education: Partners for learning. In M. A. Perez & R. R. Luquis (Eds.), *Cultural competence in health education and health promotion* (pp. 201–212). San Francisco, CA: Jossey-Bass.

Andrulis, D. P., & Brach, C. (2007). Integrating literacy, culture, and language to improve health care quality for diverse populations. *American Journal of Health Behavior, 31*(Suppl. 1), S122–S133.

Association of American Medical Colleges. (2011). *FACTS: Applicants, matriculants, enrollment, graduates, MD/PhD, and residency applicants data.* Retrieved from https://www.aamc.org/data/facts

Bennett, I. M., Chen, J., Soroui, J. S., & White, S. (2009). The contribution of health literacy to disparities in self-rated health status and preventive health behaviors in older adults. *Annals of Family Medicine, 7*(3), 204–211.

Betancourt, J. R., & Green, A. R. (2010). Linking cultural competence training to improved health outcomes: Perspectives from the field. *Academic Medicine, 85*(4), 583–585.

Betancourt, J. R., Green, A. R., & Carrillo, J. E. (2002). *Cultural competence in health care: Emerging frameworks and practical approaches.* New York, NY: The

Commonwealth Fund. Retrieved from http://www.commonwealthfund.org/usr_doc/betancourt_culturalcompetence_576.pdf

Betancourt, J. R., Green, A. R., Carrillo, J. E., & Ananeh-Firempong, O. (2003). Defining cultural competence: A practical framework for addressing racial/ethnic disparities in health and health care. *Public Health Reports, 118*(4), 293–302.

Bolin, J. N., & Bellamy, G. (2011). *Rural healthy people 2020.* College Station, TX: Texas A&M Health Science Center. Retrieved from http://cchd.us/wp-content/uploads/2015/04/ruralhealthy2020.pdf

Butler, M., Talley, K. M. C., Burns, R., Ripley, A., Rothman, A., Johnson, P., . . . Kane, R. L. (2011). *Values of older adults related to primary and secondary prevention.* Rockville, MD: Agency for Healthcare Research and Quality. Retrieved from http://www.ncbi.nlm.nih.gov/books/NBK53769

Castaneda, D. E., Organista, K. C., Rodriguez, L., & Check, P. (2013). Evaluating an entertainment–education telenovela to promote workplace safety. *Sage Open, 3*(3). doi:10.1177/21582401350028

Centers for Disease Control and Prevention. (2015a, April 28). *Minority health: Populations.* Retrieved from http://www.cdc.gov/minorityhealth

Centers for Disease Control and Prevention. (2015b, August 4). *Women's health.* Retrieved from http://www.cdc.gov/women

Center for Linguistic and Cultural Competence in Health Care, Office of Minority Health, U.S. Department of Health and Human Services. *Think Cultural Health: E-learning programs.* Retrieved from https://www.thinkculturalhealth.hhs.gov/Content/about_tch.asp

Findley, A. (2015). Low health literacy and older adults: Meanings, problems, and recommendations for social work. *Social Work in Health Care, 54*(1), 65–81.

Fitzpatrick, A. L., Steinman, L. E., Tu, S. P., Ly, K. A., Ton, T. G., Yip, M., & Sin, M. (2012). Using photovoice to understand cardiovascular health awareness in Asian elders. *Health Promotion Practice, 13*(1), 48–54.

Flora, C. B. (1980). Fotonovelas: Message creation and reception. *Journal of Popular Culture, 14*(3), 524–534.

Flores, G., Gee, D., & Kastner, B. (2000). The teaching of cultural issues in U.S. and Canadian medical schools. *Academic Medicine, 75*(5), 451–455.

Fortier, J. P., & Bishop, D. (2004). *Setting the agenda for research on cultural competence in health care: Final Report.* Edited by C. Brach, Rockville, MD: U.S. Department of Health and Human Services, Office of Minority Health and Agency for Healthcare Research and Quality.

Galambos, C. (2003). Moving cultural diversity toward cultural competence in health care. *Health & Social Work, 28*(1), 3–7.

Guy, T. C. (1999). *Providing culturally relevant adult education: A challenge for the twenty-first century.* San Francisco, CA: Jossey-Bass.

Horrell, B., Stephens, C., & Breheny, M. (2015). Capability to care: Supporting the health of informal caregivers for older people. *Health Psychology, 34*(4), 339–348.

Hsu, J. (2010). *Overview of military culture* [PowerPoint slides]. Retrieved from http://www.apa.org/about/gr/issues/military/military-culture.pdf

Keller, C., Vega-López, S., Ainsworth, B., Nagle-Williams, A., Records, K., Permana, P., & Coonrod, D. (2014). Social marketing: Approach to cultural and contextual relevance in a community-based physical activity intervention. *Health Promotion International*, *29*(1), 130–140.

Kindig, D. A., Panzer, A. M., & Nielsen-Bohlman, L. (Eds.). (2004). *Health literacy: A prescription to end confusion*. Washington, DC: National Academies Press.

Koenig, C. J., Maguen, S., Monroy, J. D., Mayott, L., & Seal, K. H. (2014). Facilitating culture-centered communication between health care providers and veterans transitioning from military deployment to civilian life. *Patient Education and Counseling*, *95*(3), 414–420.

Koh, H. K., Gracia, J. N., & Alvarez, M. E. (2014). Culturally and linguistically appropriate services: Advancing health with CLAS. *New England Journal of Medicine*, *371*(3), 198–201.

Kutner, M., Greenburg, E., Jin, Y., & Paulsen, C. (2006). *The Health Literacy of America's Adults: Results from the 2003 National Assessment of Adult Literacy*. Washington, DC: National Center for Education Statistics. Retrieved from http://files.eric .ed.gov/fulltext/ED493284.pdf

Kutob, R. M., Bormanis, J., Crago, M., Harris, J. M., Senf, J., & Shisslak, C. M. (2013). Cultural competence education for practicing physicians: Lessons in cultural humility, nonjudgmental behaviors, and health beliefs elicitation. *Journal of Continuing Education in the Health Professions*, *33*(3), 164–173.

Langer, N. (2008). Integrating compliance, communication, and culture: Delivering health care to an aging population. *Educational Gerontology*, *34*(5), 385–396.

LaViest, T., Gaskin, D., & Richard, P. (2009). *The economic burden of health inequalities in the United States*. Washington, DC: Joint Center for Political and Economic Studies.

Levin, J., Chatters, L. M., & Taylor, R. J. (2005). Religion, health and medicine in African Americans: Implications for physicians. *Journal of the National Medical Association*, *97*(2), 237–249.

Lie, D., Carter-Pokras, O., Braun, B., & Coleman, C. (2012). What do health literacy and cultural competence have in common? Calling for a collaborative health professional pedagogy. *Journal of Health Communication*, *17*(3), 13–22.

Logan, R. A., Wong, W. F., Villaire, M., Daus, G., Parnell, T. A., Willis, E., & Paasche-Orlow, M. K. (2015). *Health literacy: A necessary element for achieving health equity*. Discussion Paper, Washington, DC: Institute of Medicine. Retrieved from http:// nam.edu/wp-content/uploads/2015/07/NecessaryElement.pdf

Lyons, B. P., Dunson-Strane, T., & Sherman, F. T. (2014). The joys of caring for older adults: Training practitioners to empower older adults. *Journal of Community Health*, *39*(3), 464–470.

Manafo, E., & Wong, S. (2012). Health literacy programs for older adults: A systematic literature review. *Health Education Research*, *27*(6), 947–960.

Meit, M. (2004). *Bridging the health divide: The rural public health research agenda*. Bradford, PA: University of Pittsburgh Center for Rural Health Practice. Retrieved from https://www.upb.pitt.edu/uploadedFiles/About/Sponsored_Programs/ Center_for_Rural_Health_Practice/Bridging%20the%20Health%20Divide.pdf

National Center for Cultural Competence. *The compelling need for cultural and linguistic competence*. Retrieved from http://nccc.georgetown.edu/foundations/ need.html

Office of Disease Prevention and Health Promotion, U.S. Department of Health and Human Services. (2010). *National action plan to improve health literacy.* Retrieved from http://www.health.gov/communication/hlactionplan/pdf/Health_Literacy_Action_Plan.pdf

Office of Minority Health, U.S. Department of Health and Human Services. *The National CLAS Standards.* Retrieved from http://minorityhealth.hhs.gov/omh/browse.aspx?lvl=2&lvlid=53

Orem, R. A. (2005). *Teaching adult English language learners.* Malabar, FL: Krieger.

Osborne, H. (2012). *Health literacy from A to Z.* Sudbury, MA: Jones & Bartlett.

Ownby, R. L., Waldrop-Valverde, D., & Taha, J. (2012). Why is health literacy related to health? An exploration among U.S. National Assessment of Adult Literacy participants 40 years of age and older. *Educational Gerontology, 38*(11), 776–787.

Parker, R. M., Williams, M. V, Weiss, B. D., Baker, D. W., Davis, T. C., Doak, C. C., & Somers, S. A. (1999). Health literacy: Report of the council on scientific affairs. *Journal of the American Medical Association, 281*(6), 552–557.

Plain Writing Act of 2010, Public Law No. 111-274, 5 USC § 301, 124 Stat. 2861 (2010). Retrieved from http://www.gpo.gov/fdsys/pkg/PLAW-111publ274/pdf/PLAW-111publ274.pdf

Purdie, N., & McCrindle, A. (2002). Self-regulation, self-efficacy and health behavior change in older adults. *Educational Gerontology, 28*(5), 379–400.

Rubin, D. (2014). Applied linguistics as a resource for understanding and advancing health literacy. In H. E. Hamilton & W. S. Chou (Eds.), *The Routledge handbook of language and health communication* (pp. 153–167). New York, NY: Routledge.

Speros, C. (2009). More than words: Promoting health literacy in older adults. *Online Journal of Issues in Nursing, 14*(3). doi:10.3912/OJIN.Vol14No03Mar5

Tufte, R. (2009). *Telenovelas, culture and social change: From polisemy, pleasure and resistance to strategic communication and social development.* Retrieved from http://www.portalcomunicacion.com/catunesco/download/tufte_telenovelas.pdf

U.S. Census Bureau. Retrieved from http://www.census.gov

Valle, R., Yamada, A. M., & Matiella, A. C. (2006). Fotonovelas: A health literacy tool for educating Latino older adults about dementia. *Clinical Gerontologist, 30*(1), 71–88.

Whaley, B. B. (Ed.). (2000). *Explaining illness: Research theory and strategies.* Mahwah, NJ: Lawrence Erlbaum.

Yeo, G. (2009). How will the U.S. healthcare system meet the challenge of the ethnogeriatric imperative? *Journal of the American Geriatrics Society, 57*(7), 1278–1285.

Young, D., Weinert, C., & Spring, A. (2012). Home on the range: Health literacy, rural elderly, well-being. *Journal of Extension, 50*(3), 3FEA2.

Zamora, H., & Clingerman, E. (2011). Health literacy among older adults: A systematic literature review. *Journal of Gerontological Nursing, 37*(10), 41–51.

Ziegahn, L., & Ton, H. (2011). Adult educators and cultural competence within health care systems: Change at the individual and structural levels. *New Directions for Adult and Continuing Education, 130,* 55–64.

CHAPTER 13

Physical Activity and Exercise for the Aging Population

TOMMIE CHURCH

With the increasing numbers of older adults (65 and older) in the United States, focus on reducing the prevalence of chronic disease and associated risk factors is essential. Currently, adults 65 years and older make up 13% of the U.S. population, and it is predicted that within 25 years, they will make up 20% of the population (American Psychological Association, 2015). In fact, by 2030, it is estimated that the number of individuals 65 years and older will reach 71 million. Currently, the average life expectancy for men and women aged 65 is 17.9 years and 20.5 years, respectively. This means that average life span for both men and women exceeds 82 years of age (Centers for Disease Control and Prevention [CDC], 2015a). Unfortunately, average healthy life span for individuals in the United States at age 65 is 12.9 for males and 14.8 years for females (CDC, 2015b). The most common causes of death in individuals 65 and older are heart disease, cancer, and chronic lower respiratory disease. These are chronic diseases with modifiable risk factors that include physical inactivity, smoking, obesity, diabetes, and hypertension. The percentage of persons 65 and older who smoke is 8.8%. The percentage of men aged 65 to 74 who are obese is 36.4%, while the percentage for ages 75 and above is 27.4%. For women, the percentages are 44.2% and 29.8% for ages 65 to 74 and 75 and older, respectively. The percentage of noninstitutionalized persons aged 65 and older with diabetes is 28.5%. The percentage of males aged 65 to 74 with hypertension is 61.7%, while the percentage of males aged 75 and older with hypertension is 75.1%. The percentage of women aged 65 to 74 with hypertension is 66.7% and the percentage of those aged 75 and older with hypertension is 79.3% (CDC, 2015a).

In the United States, the cost of health care associated with chronic conditions and diseases is exorbitant. In 2006, 84% of the total health care spending was for the 50% of the population in the United States who suffered from chronic conditions. The total costs for heart disease and stroke in 2010 were estimated at $315.4 billion. Cancer treatment represented $157 billion in 2010, while diagnosed diabetes represented total medical costs of $245 billion in 2012. Furthermore, it is estimated that physical inactivity causes 6% of the burden of coronary heart disease, 7% of type 2 diabetes, and 10% of breast and colon cancer cases worldwide (Exercise Is Medicine, 2015).

By increasing physical activity of individuals in the United States, it is possible to reduce risk for many of these chronic conditions. Physical activity can also serve as treatment for chronic conditions such as arthritis, heart disease, and diabetes. Additionally, regular physical activity is essential for healthy aging. It enables individuals to continue to be able to carry out activities of daily living (ADLs) and maintain independent living. Regular physical activity can improve mental health, balance, and bone health (National Institute on Aging, 2014). Participation in regular physical activity has been shown to be effective in reducing the functional decline that is associated with aging. More specifically, aerobic training can maintain and improve various aspects of heart and lung function, while resistance training can help offset muscle and strength losses, typical during aging, which can improve functional movement capacity.

WHAT IS PHYSICAL ACTIVITY?

Physical activity can be defined as "movement produced by skeletal muscle that results in energy expenditure" (World Health Organization, 2015). Physical activity can include a variety of activities including occupational work, household chores, sports, leisure activity, and exercise.

"Exercise" is a subset of physical activity that is planned, structured, and repeated with the intent of maintaining or improving physical fitness (Insel & Roth, 2012).

WHAT IS PHYSICAL FITNESS?

"Physical fitness" is the ability of the body to respond or adapt to the demands and stress of physical effort (Insel & Roth, 2012). There are two types of physical fitness: skill-related and health-related fitness. Skill-related fitness components include agility, balance, coordination, power, reaction time, and speed. These attributes are important when participating in a variety of sports. Health-related components include cardiorespiratory endurance, muscular strength, muscular endurance, flexibility, and body composition. Exercise programs typically include planned activities that focus on health-related fitness components and each of these are associated with a variety of benefits to overall health and quality of life. The focus of this chapter will be on health-related fitness and how physical activity and exercise focusing on health-related fitness benefit adults aged 65 years and older related to health status and quality of life.

Health-Related Physical Fitness Components

"Cardiorespiratory endurance" can be defined as "the ability of the circulatory and respiratory systems to supply oxygen during sustained physical activity" (American College of Sports Medicine [ACSM], 2014a). Cardiorespiratory activities, also referred to as "aerobic activities," help make the heart and lungs stronger and the circulatory system more efficient. Some of the activities that can be used to improve cardiorespiratory endurance include bicycling, walking, jogging, swimming, raking leaves, sweeping the floor, dancing, and playing tennis (National Institute on Aging, 2014). Maximum oxygen uptake (VO_2max) is the most commonly used measure of cardiorespiratory endurance and can be defined as "the maximum volume of oxygen that can be utilized in 1 minute during maximal or exhaustive exercise. It is measured in milliliters of oxygen used in 1 minute per kilogram of body of weight" (Quinn, 2016). Research findings indicate that VO_2max decreases 5% to 15% per decade beginning at 25 to 30 years of age. This can be offset by participating in aerobic training. According to ACSM (2015), the same 10% to 30% increases in VO_2max that can be achieved by young adults who participate in aerobic training can also occur in older adults who participate in aerobic training.

"Muscular strength" can be defined as "the ability of a muscle or group of muscles to exert force" (ACSM, 2014).

"Muscular endurance" can be defined as "the ability of muscle to continue to perform without fatigue" (ACSM, 2014). Some of the types of activities that improve muscular strength and endurance are resistance training, calisthenics, and group exercise programs like Pilates, yoga, and tai chi. Muscular strength and endurance activities are important for the aging individual because they make it easier to carry out ADLs such as getting up from a chair, climbing stairs, carrying groceries, opening jars, and improving balance capabilities. Also, resistance training can reduce muscle mass loss that is typically associated with aging. Additional benefits include reduced risk of osteoporosis, improved postural stability, reduced risk of falls, and better mobility in general (ACSM, 2014b).

In addition to muscular fitness exercises, balance exercises can also reduce risk of falls, and consequent fractures. Examples of exercises for improving balance include backward walking, sideways walking, heel and toe walking, and standing from sitting position. These activities can increase in difficulty by progressing from using support while executing movement to using no support while executing movement.

"Flexibility" can be defined as "the range of motion available at a joint" (ACSM, 2014). Since flexibility is joint specific, an individual can have optimal flexibility in some joints and very poor flexibility in others. Exercise training with stretching exercises and programs like martial arts, Pilates, and yoga help maintain and/or improve range of motion and allow for continuance of ADLs like dressing and reaching for items on a shelf. Even though recent studies question the benefits of stretching to prevent injury and delayed-onset muscle soreness, flexibility training can be used by older adults to maintain the range of motion needed to maintain functional capacity. (ACSM, 2014b) suggests slow easy stretches at the end of exercise sessions to offset the lack of elasticity in older adults' muscles.

"Body composition" can be defined as "relative amounts of muscle, fat, bone, and other vital parts of the body" (ACSM, 2014). Even though older adults may maintain the same body weight, sarcopenia (muscle loss) and increases in body fat are typical changes that occur in aging adults. Additionally, increased fat mass is distributed more specifically to the abdominal area, which is associated with increased risk of cardiovascular disease and diabetes. Exercise training that includes resistance training and weight-bearing aerobic activity can help offset changes in body composition that typically occur with aging (St. Onge & Gallagher, 2010).

HOW ACTIVE ARE OLDER ADULTS?

Even though research evidences the negative impact of inactivity on health and conversely, the benefits of being more physically active throughout the life span, midlife and older adults are the most inactive of all age groups of the population. According to the President's Council on Physical Fitness, Sports, and Nutrition (2014), only 28% to 34% of adults aged 65 to 74 are physically active, and 35% to 44% of adults aged 75 and older are physically active. In all age groups, less than 5% of adults participate in 30 minutes of physical activity each day, and only one in three adults get the recommended amount of physical activity each week. Additionally, 80% of adults do not meet the guidelines for both aerobic and muscle-strengthening activities.

WHAT ARE THE GENERAL PRINCIPLES OF EXERCISE TRAINING?

The principle of overload states that in order to continue to reap benefits with an exercise program, an individual must continue to stress the body more than is usual. This causes the body systems that are stressed during activity to adapt. It is important to make small progressive increases that result in safe continued overload of the body systems. This can be accomplished by increasing one or more of the following: frequency, intensity, or duration. Utilizing overload in aerobic activity can result in improvements in the efficiency and capacity of the heart, lungs, circulatory system, and working muscles. Muscle and bone-strengthening activities can overload muscles and bones and result in strength gains in them (USA Triathlon, 2015).

The principle of specificity means that the body systems that are overloaded during physical activity or exercise are the ones that reap the benefits. It is important to select the appropriate types of activity to reap the desired benefits. For example, aerobic activity benefits the heart, lungs, and circulatory system while resistance training benefits the body by strengthening muscles and bones (USA Triathlon, 2015).

The principle of adaptation means that the body adapts to exercise training gradually over time, and this adaptation results in better efficiency and less effort required over time (USA Triathlon, 2015).

Individual differences states that everyone has different responses to exercise based on a variety of factors including genetics, previous experience, nutrition, environment, rest, stress, and motivation (USA Triathlon, 2015). For this reason, exercise programs should be tailored to each individual's needs, goals, and limitations.

The principle of reversibility, also referred to as the "use it or lose it" principle, states that regular exercise is required for adaptation to occur and be maintained. If an individual ceases an exercise program, the result, over time, will be a loss of the positive adaptations gained during the exercise program (USA Triathlon, 2015).

The FITT principle includes frequency, intensity, time, and type. One or more of these components are increased to implement overload. Every exercise prescription includes frequency, intensity, time, and type.

Frequency—how many days per week a person exercises.

Intensity—effort required to participate in activity. Methods of measuring intensity vary depending on the type of exercise. Time/duration refers to the length of time for each exercise session. Type/mode refers to the specific type of activity used in the exercise session.

FITT Principle for Improving Cardiorespiratory Endurance in Apparently Healthy Adults

Frequency of 3 to 5 days per week promotes improvement. Beginners should start with 3 days per week working toward 5 days per week.

Intensity can be expressed in terms of metabolic units (METs), VO_2 (mL/kg/min), percentage of maximum heart rate, or rate of perceived exertion (RPE). Two of the most common ways for an individual to monitor intensity during an exercise session are by monitoring heart rate or using the talk test.

To achieve cardiorespiratory benefits, a target heart rate zone of 50% to 90% of maximum heart rate is suggested (CDC, 2014). To calculate target heart rate zones for moderate intensity, the first step is to determine the person's age-related maximum heart rate by subtracting the individual's age from 220. For example, if a person is 70 years old, the estimated maximum heart rate would be 150 beats per minute. To determine moderate intensity heart rate zone, 50% to 70% maximum heart rate:

- 50% level = 150 × 0.50 = 75 bpm
- 70% level = 150 × 0.70 = 105 bpm

To determine vigorous intensity heart rate zone, 70% to 85% maximum heart rate:

- 70% level = 150 × 0.70 = 105 bpm
- 85% level = 150 × 0.85 = 127.5 or approximately 128 bpm

When monitoring intensity using the heart rate method during exercise, the individual must stop briefly to palpate pulse. Pulse can be taken at the wrist (radial pulse) or at the neck (carotid). By taking pulse for only 15 seconds and multiplying by four to determine per minute rate, the individual has to stop only briefly to determine if intensity will benefit cardiorespiratory endurance.

The "talk test" is a simpler method of monitoring intensity during exercise and requires the participant to monitor breathing. During moderately intense activity, the individual should have some mild shortness of breath, dyspnea, during activity but should still be able to talk.

Absolute intensity is the measure of energy expenditure per minute. Absolute intensity can be expressed in terms of METs, milliliters of oxygen per kilogram weight per minute, or calories per minute. Without specialized equipment, these measures are not available to the exercise participant. However, examples of moderate and vigorous intensities are represented in Tables 13.1 and 13.2.

Time for cardiorespiratory endurance training in apparently healthy adults is 20 to 60 minutes per day in sessions lasting at least 10 minutes each.

Type of exercise for cardiorespiratory endurance training includes rhythmic activities that utilize the large muscle groups of the body.

TABLE 13.1 Moderate Intensity Cardiorespiratory (Aerobic) Activities

- Walking briskly (3 mph or faster but not race walk)
- Water aerobics
- Bicycling slower than 10 mph
- Tennis (doubles)
- Ballroom dancing
- General gardening

Source: CDC (2015d).

TABLE 13.2 Vigorous Intensity Cardiorespiratory (Aerobic) Activities

- Race walking, jogging, or running
- Swimming laps
- Tennis (singles)
- Aerobic dancing
- Bicycling 10 miles per hour or faster
- Jumping rope
- Heavy gardening (continuous digging or hoeing)
- Hiking uphill or with a heavy backpack

Source: CDC (2015d).

Aerobic activity is synonymous with "Cardiorespiratory"; activity in which the body keeps up the oxygen supply needed for large muscle activity.

FITT Principle for Improving Muscular Strength in Apparently Healthy Adults

Frequency for improving muscular strength includes at least 2 non-consecutive days.

Intensity for muscular strength improvement includes sufficient weight load to fatigue muscles.

Time for muscular strength improvement includes one or more sets of 8 to 12 repetitions.

Type includes resistance exercises for all of the major muscle groups.

FITT Principle for Improving Flexibility in Apparently Healthy Adults

Frequency is at least 2 to 3 days per week.

Intensity includes stretching to the point of discomfort.

Time includes two to four repetitions of each exercise, for 15 to 30 seconds each.

Type includes stretching exercises utilizing all the major muscle groups.

WHAT ARE THE GENERAL GUIDELINES FOR PHYSICAL ACTIVITY FOR OLDER ADULTS?

- At least 2.5 hours (150 minutes) of moderately intense aerobic activity (i.e., brisk walking) every week
- 2 or more days of muscular strengthening activities (major muscle groups: legs, hips, back, abdomen, chest, shoulders, and arms)—resistance training with weight machines or free weights; calisthenics that use body as resistance (push-ups and crunches); heavy gardening, yoga
- 75 minutes per week of vigorous intensity aerobic activities (i.e., jogging or running)
- 2 or more days of muscle strengthening activities using the major muscle groups of the body (legs, hips, back, abdomen, chest, shoulders, and arms)

For greater health benefits, older adults can increase their activity level to:

- 5 hours (300 minutes) of moderately intense aerobic activities each week
- Same regimen as above of muscle strengthening activities

Or

- 2.5 hours (150 minutes) of vigorous aerobic activities per week
- Same regimen of muscle strengthening activities

WHAT ARE THE HEALTH BENEFITS OF BEING PHYSICALLY ACTIVE?

In addition to maintaining or increasing health-related physical fitness, the health benefits of physical activity for adults and older adults include:

Strong Evidence
- Lower risk of premature death
- Lower risk of coronary heart disease
- Lower risk of stroke
- Lower risk of high blood pressure
- Lower risk of adverse blood lipid (cholesterol) profile
- Lower risk of type 2 diabetes
- Lower risk of metabolic syndrome
- Lower risk of colon cancer
- Lower risk of breast cancer
- Prevention of weight gain
- Weight loss when combined with reduced calorie intake
- Prevention of falls
- Reduced depression
- Better cognitive function (older adults)

Moderate to strong evidence
- Better functional health (older adults)
- Reduced abdominal obesity

Moderate evidence
- Lower risk of hip fracture
- Lower risk of lung cancer
- Lower risk of endometrial cancer
- Weight maintenance after weight loss

- Increased bone density
- Improved sleep quality

Source: Office of Disease Prevention and Health Promotion, (2015a).

HOW MUCH ACTIVITY IS REQUIRED TO GET HEALTH BENEFITS?

Lower Premature Death Risk

People who participate in physical activity for 7 hours per week are estimated to have 40% lower risk of dying prematurely compared to those who are active for less than 30 minutes a week. However, even those who participate in moderately intense activity for just 150 minutes (2.5 hours) have lowered risk for premature death, and so do those who are active for just 90 minutes; therefore, some activity is better than no activity in reducing risks for premature death (Office of Disease Prevention and Health Promotion, 2015a).

Cardiovascular Health

People who participate in moderate aerobic physical activity for at least 150 minutes per week have significant reduction in risk for cardiovascular disease, with greater benefits occurring with 200 minutes a week. There is strong evidence that greater amounts of physical activity result in greater reductions in the risk of cardiovascular disease (Office of Disease Prevention and Health Promotion, 2015a).

Metabolic Health

"Metabolic syndrome" is defined as a condition in which people have some combination of high blood pressure, abdominal obesity, an adverse blood lipid profile (abnormal cholesterol or triglycerides), and impaired blood glucose tolerance. Participating in at least moderate physical activity for 120 to 150 minutes per week can reduce risks of having metabolic syndrome with greater benefits resulting from an increase in activity levels (Office of Disease Prevention and Health Promotion, 2015a).

Individuals with diabetes can reduce their risk for heart disease by participating in physical activity. Participating in 150 minutes per week of moderately intense aerobic activity can lower risks, while increasing to 300 minutes per week can produce greater benefits. However, individuals with diabetes should consult their health care provider before beginning an activity program to make sure the planned activity is appropriate for their condition and to discuss the monitoring of blood glucose and avoidance of injury to their feet (Office of Disease Prevention and Health Promotion, 2015a).

Obesity and Energy Balance

Physical activity helps individuals maintain weight, but the optimal amount needed to maintain weight varies among people. However, people who participate in 150 to 300 minutes of activity equivalent in intensity to a 4 mile per hour walking pace can maintain weight over a short period of time, such as a year. People who want to lose more than 5% of their body weight may need to participate in more than 300 minutes of moderate-intensity activity per week (Office of Disease Prevention and Health Promotion, 2015a).

Musculoskeletal Health

Maintaining muscle, bone, and joint health is important as people age. Bone density reduction that occurs during the aging process can be slowed with regular physical activity as can muscle atrophy. People who participate in aerobic, muscle-strengthening, and bone-strengthening activities can slow down bone density loss with 90 to 300 minutes of physical activity. Additionally, those who participate in 120 to 300 minutes of moderate-intensity physical activity reduce their risk for hip fractures.

Progressive muscle-strengthening activities increase or maintain muscle mass, strength, and power. Resistance training also improves muscular strength in individuals with conditions like multiple sclerosis, stroke, and spinal cord injury. Even though aerobic activity doesn't increase muscle mass in the same way that resistance training does, it may also slow the loss of muscle that occurs during the aging process (Office of Disease Prevention and Health Promotion, 2015a).

Osteoarthritis can cause pain and fatigue. This may make it difficult for those with this chronic condition to start or continue to be physically active. However, done safely, regular physical activity does not make the disease or pain worse. Aerobic activity and muscular strength-building activities can result in pain reduction and improve physical function, quality of life, and mental health (Office of Disease Prevention and Health Promotion, 2015a).

Osteoporosis is a disease that results in loss of bone density and poor bone strength. Any type of weight-bearing exercise, including walking, jogging, and resistance training can help maintain bone density throughout an individual's life span. With stronger bones and muscles, there is reduced risk for falls and fractures (Insel & Roth, 2012).

Functional Ability and Fall Prevention

Functional ability is the ability of individuals to carry out ADLs such as climbing stairs, walking on sidewalk, personal care, grocery shopping, playing with grandchildren, and so forth. Although unclear about the amount of exercise needed for maintaining or improving functional ability, it is important to include both aerobic and muscle-strengthening physical activity to ensure maintenance of functional ability. Reduction in falls has been seen in individuals who participate in at least 90 minutes of balance and muscle-strengthening activities coupled with at least 60 minutes of moderate-intensity walking per week (Office of Disease Prevention and Health Promotion, 2015a).

Cancer

Research shows that a variety of moderate-intensity physical activity for 210 to 420 minutes a week is needed to significantly reduce the risk of colon and breast cancer. Lower amounts (i.e., 150 minutes per week) do not appear to provide major benefits in this aspect of disease prevention. Cancer survivors should participate in physical activity to help reduce the risk of new chronic diseases. Studies suggest that individuals with colon or breast cancer who are physically active are less likely to die prematurely or have a reoccurrence of the cancer. Physical activity may also help reduce the side effects of cancer treatment. As with other chronic conditions, cancer survivors should consult their health care provider to make sure the planned activity is appropriate for their condition and health status (Office of Disease Prevention and Health Promotion, 2015a).

Mental Health

Adults who participate regularly in physical activity have a lower risk of depression and cognitive decline. These benefits have been found in individuals who participate in a combination of aerobic and muscle strengthening physical activities 3 to 5 days per week for 30 to 60 minutes' duration for each session (Office of Disease Prevention and Health Promotion, 2015a).

WHAT ARE THE STEPS THAT OLDER ADULTS NEED TO TAKE TO GET STARTED WITH AN EXERCISE PROGRAM?

Prescreening and Medical Clearance

According to ACSM (2014), an extensive medical examination is not necessary for apparently healthy individuals who plan to begin a light- to moderate-intensity physical activity program. However, ACSM does recommend a risk stratification approach to starting an exercise program. Factors that are used to stratify risks include age, high blood pressure, abnormal cholesterol levels, and family history of heart disease, smoking habit, obesity, and abnormal glucose tolerance. At the very least, an adult planning to begin an exercise program should complete a self-administered screening tool like the Physical Activity Readiness Questionnaire (PAR-Q) or the AHA/ACSM Health/Fitness Facility Pre-Participation Questionnaire. (See sample questions for both of these instruments in Boxes 13.1 and 13.2.). Results from this type of questionnaire will suggest whether medical clearance and/or exercise testing is recommended prior to beginning an exercise program.

BOX 13.1 Physical Activity Readiness Questionnaire

1. Has your doctor ever said that you have a heart condition and that you should do physical activity only when recommended by a doctor?
2. Do you feel pain in your chest when you do physical activity?
3. In the past month, have you had chest pain when you were not doing physical activity?
4. Do you lose your balance because of dizziness or do you ever lose consciousness?
5. Do you have a bone or joint problem (e.g., back, knee, or hip) that could be made worse by a change in your physical activity?
6. Is your doctor currently prescribing drugs (e.g., water pills) for your blood pressure or heart condition?
7. Do you know of any other reason why you should not do physical activity?

If you answered yes to one or more of these questions, see your doctor before you start becoming much more physically active or before you have a fitness appraisal.

Source: ACSM (2014a).

BOX 13.2 AHA/ACSM Health/Fitness Facility Preparticipation Screening Questionnaire

Assess Your Health Needs by Marking All True Statements.
HISTORY
You have had:
    A heart attack
    Heart surgery
    Cardiac catheterization
    Coronary angioplasty (percutaneous transluminal coronary angioplasty [PTCA])
    Pacemaker/implantable cardiac defibrillator/rhythm disturbance
    Heart valve disease
    Heart failure
    Heart transplantation
    Congenital heart disease
SYMPTOMS
    You experience chest discomfort with exertion.
    You experience unreasonable breathlessness.
    You experience dizziness, fainting, and blackouts.
    You take heart medications.
OTHER HEALTH ISSUES
    You have musculoskeletal problems.
    You have concerns about the safety of exercise.
    You take prescription medication(s).
    You are pregnant.
If you marked any of the statements in this section, consult your
  health care provider before engaging in exercise. You may need to
  use a facility with a medically qualified staff.

CARDIOVASCULAR RISK FACTORS
    You are a man older than 45 years.
    You are a woman older than 55 years or you have had a hysterectomy or you are postmenopausal.
    You smoke.
    Your blood pressure is greater than 140/90.
    You don't know your blood pressure.
    You take blood pressure medication.

(continued)

BOX 13.2 AHA/ACSM Health/Fitness Facility Preparticipation Screening Questionnaire (*continued*)

Your blood cholesterol level is greater than 240 mg/dL.
You don't know your cholesterol level.
You have a close blood relative who had a heart attack before age 55 (father or brother) or age 65 (mother or sister).
You are physically inactive (i.e., you get less than 30 minutes of physical activity on at least 3 days per week).
You are greater than 20 pounds overweight.

If you marked two or more of the statements in this section, consult your health care provider before engaging in exercise. You might benefit by using a facility with a professionally qualified exercise staff to guide your exercise program.

None of the above is true.
You should be able to exercise safely without consulting your health care provider in almost any facility that meets your exercise program needs.

Source: ACSM (2014a).

WHO NEEDS MEDICAL CLEARANCE?

Individuals who have no more than one risk factor for cardiovascular, pulmonary, or metabolic disease are stratified as low risk and medical clearance is not necessary for these individuals regardless of whether initiating a light, moderate, or vigorous exercise program. Individuals who have two or more risk factors for cardiovascular, pulmonary, or metabolic disease are stratified as moderate risk for cardiac events during exercise and are encouraged to consult their physician prior to starting a vigorous exercise program. Medical clearance is not necessary if they are starting a light-moderate intensity exercise program like walking. Individuals with symptoms or diagnosed cardiovascular, pulmonary, or metabolic disease are stratified as high risk and should consult with their physician before beginning any exercise program.

TABLE 13.3 Risk Stratification

Low to Moderate Risk
- Fasting total serum cholesterol, LDL cholesterol, HDL cholesterol, and triglycerides
- Fasting plasma glucose
- Thyroid function, if abnormal cholesterol is present

High Risk
- Same tests as those for low and moderate risk
- 12-lead ECG, holter monitoring, coronary angiography, radionuclide or echocardiograph studies
- Carotid ultrasound and other peripheral vascular studies
- Chest radiograph (individuals with suspected or present heart failure)
- Comprehensive blood chemistry panel and blood count

Patients With Pulmonary Disease
- Chest radiograph
- Pulmonary function tests
- Carbon dioxide diffusing capacity
- Other specialized pulmonary studies such as blood gas analysis

Source: ACSM (2014a).

WHAT LAB TESTS SHOULD BE INCLUDED WITH THE PHYSICAL EXAMINATION FOR MEDICAL CLEARANCE?

Those who are recommended to get medical clearance prior to initiating an exercise program should receive a physical exam by a physician or other qualified health care provider. Lab tests that should be included as per risk stratification level are included in Table 13.3.

WHAT ARE RECOMMENDATIONS FOR EXERCISE TESTING PRIOR TO BEGINNING AN EXERCISE PROGRAM?

Graded exercise testing is routinely recommended for only those individuals who are stratified as high risk. One of the purposes of administering exercise testing to high risk individuals is to determine risks of cardiac events with exercise. Exercise testing by a nonphysician health care provider or professional specially trained in clinical exercise testing is permissible for individuals of low, moderate, and high risk without a physician present, but immediately available if needed. Physicians who supervise exercise testing should, at minimum, meet the competencies established by the American Heart Association for supervision and interpretation of exercise tests. Also, one or more of the professionals administering the exercise test should at least have cardiopulmonary resuscitation (CPR) certification and automated defibrillator (AED) training. Preferably, one or more of the staff should also have advanced cardiac life support (ACLS) certification. Individuals who are stratified as low risk do not need a physician immediately available. Even though exercise testing is not always recommended for those with low to moderate risk, it can provide important information for designing a safe and effective exercise prescription for individuals of any risk stratification.

HOW PREVALENT ARE CARDIAC RISKS DURING EXERCISE TESTING AND EXERCISE IN GENERAL?

The risk for cardiac events during exercise testing varies depending on the presence of diagnosed or hidden cardiovascular disease. Estimated risk of cardiac events during exercise testing is approximately six per 10,000 tests (ACSM, 2014). The risk of myocardial infarction (MI) or sudden cardiac death occurring during exercise is definitely higher in older adults than their younger counterparts due to the higher prevalence of cardiovascular disease (CVD) in older adults. According to ACSM (2014), the risk of sudden cardiac death during vigorous intensity exercise is estimated at one per year for every 15,000 to 18,000 individuals who had been asymptomatic prior to exercising. Additionally, risks for MI and sudden cardiac death are even higher for sedentary individuals who perform unaccustomed exercise or infrequent exercise. Consequently, even though there is increased risk for cardiac events with vigorous intensity exercise, individuals who are physically active have approximately 30% to 40% lower risk of developing CVD than those who are inactive (ACSM, 2014).

WHAT ARE THE CONTRAINDICATIONS TO EXERCISE TESTING?

For some individuals, the potential risks of exercise testing outweigh the benefits. Individuals with absolute contraindications to exercise should avoid exercise testing until conditions are stabilized or adequately treated. Individuals with relative contraindications should be tested only after a careful benefit-risk evaluation has been conducted (ACSM, 2014). A sample of the absolute and relative contraindications is included in

TABLE 13.4 Contraindications to Exercise Testing

Absolute
- Unstable angina
- Uncontrolled cardiac dysrhythmias
- Uncontrolled symptomatic heart failure
- Acute myocarditis or pericarditis

Relative
- Left main coronary stenosis
- Electrolyte abnormalities
- Hypertrophic cardiomyopathy
- Ventricular aneurysm

Source: ACSM (2014a).

Table 13.4. A more comprehensive list of the absolute and relative contraindications to testing is available in *ACSM's Guidelines for Exercise Testing and Prescription* (9th edition).

WHAT ARE SUGGESTED ACTIVITIES FOR INDIVIDUALS WITH STABLE MEDICAL CONDITIONS FOLLOWING MEDICAL CLEARANCE?

According to the National Council on Aging, the following activities are suggested for individuals with the following stable conditions and diseases (see Table 13.5).

WHAT ARE THE ADVANTAGES OF MEDICALLY SUPERVISED PROGRAMS POSTCARDIAC EVENT OR POSTSTROKE?

Cardiac rehabilitation is a medically supervised program that includes exercise training, education on heart healthy living, and counseling on how to reduce stress upon returning to active life following a heart attack, being diagnosed with coronary artery disease, or following various procedures or surgeries including coronary bypass graft surgery, valve replacement, implantable cardioverter defibrillator, or percutaneous coronary interventions like stenting or angioplasty. The cardiac

TABLE 13.5 Suggested Activities for Specific Stable Conditions and Diseases

Known clinical problem or symptoms	Exercise Options
Known cardiovascular disease such as high blood pressure or congestive heart failure	Progressive activity as tolerated: ▪ Walking at a comfortable pace for increasing distances ▪ Resistance training at a comfortable level, increasing intensity as tolerated ▪ Balance and flexibility exercises
Vertigo or balance problems from strength and musculoskeletal changes	Progressive activity as tolerated: ▪ Start with stepping while seated ▪ Progress to walking at a comfortable pace for increasing distances ▪ Resistance training at a comfortable level, increasing as tolerated ▪ Balance and flexibility exercises ▪ Try to have another person present during exercise activity ▪ Emphasize balance and lower body strength exercises
Degenerative joint disease, spinal stenosis, or spinal compression	▪ Avoid exercise programs that are specifically geared to walking on a hard surface ▪ Avoid resistance exercise activities (lifting weights or using resistance bands) that increase pain ▪ Pool exercise programs, or using appropriate exercise equipment to strengthen muscles surrounding sore joints ▪ Balance and flexibility exercises
Chronic obstructive pulmonary disease	▪ Walking at a comfortable pace for increasing distances ▪ Resistance training at a comfortable level, increasing intensity as tolerated ▪ Balance and flexibility exercises

Source: National Institute of Aging (2014).

rehabilitation team may include doctors, nurses, exercise specialists, physical and occupational therapists, dietitians or nutritionists, and psychologists, or other mental health specialists (National Heart, Lung, and Blood Institute, 2013).

The program begins with a medical evaluation to determine the patient's needs and limitations. Exercise training may start in a group setting in which the patient may work with a physical therapist, an exercise physiologist, and/or health care professionals who monitor heart rate and blood pressure during physical activity. A cardiac rehabilitation plan varies in duration depending on each individual patient's needs. A typical exercise program includes aerobic, strength building, and flexibility exercises. With an emphasis on improvements in cardiovascular health, the typical program may consist of 3 to 5 days of aerobic exercises for 20 to 45 minutes each session. Intermittent sessions of 10 minutes each may be used with entry level patients. Muscular strength activities typically consist of resistance training utilizing free weights, weight machines, and/or resistance bands. Static stretching at the end of each session can aid in promotion of better range of motion. General overload guidelines for strength and flexibility building are recommended, but resistance training should begin with higher repetitions and reduced weight loads.

Cardiac rehabilitation programs can last from 6 weeks up to 6 months or longer. Since physical activity reduces the chances of future heart problems, including heart attack, and also helps strengthen the heart and the rest of the body, it is definitely a beneficial program.

Benefits of cardiac rehabilitation include:

- Reduced risk of mortality, reduced risk of future heart attack
- Decreased pain
- Possible reduced need for some heart disease medicines
- Reduction of cardiovascular risk factors (e.g., blood pressure and cholesterol)
- Improved quality of life and functional capacity
- Stress reduction and improved general emotional health

Factors to consider when selecting a cardiac rehabilitation program include time the program is offered, place, services, setting, and cost. One of the main concerns of those deciding on a cardiac rehabilitation program is whether the program is covered by their health insurance plan or Medicare (National Heart, Lung, and Blood Institute, 2013).

In the past, physical rehabilitation programs for stroke survivors lasted only a few months because it was believed that most or all of the recovery of motor function occurred during this time span. However, recent studies have shown that extended rehabilitation that includes treadmill exercise, with or without weight support, can increase aerobic capacity and sensorimotor function. In addition to exercise prescriptions to improve cardiorespiratory fitness and improve motor performance, other goals of rehabilitation include improvement of self-care skills and occupational skills.

The three main goals of poststroke physical rehabilitation are to prevent the complications of prolonged inactivity, decrease risk for recurrent stroke and cardiovascular events, and increase cardiorespiratory fitness. To achieve the first goal, early initiation of activity poststroke is important. This begins with standing from sitting during hospital convalescence to remedial gait retraining, supervised home walking, and treadmill training. The second goal of reducing recurrent stroke and other cardiovascular events requires the reduction of risks for those events. An aerobic exercise program can help lower blood pressure, total blood cholesterol, triglycerides, and low-density lipoprotein cholesterol. It also can enhance blood glucose tolerance and reduce body fat stores. By controlling these risk factors, there is reduced risk for the recurrence of future strokes and cardiovascular events. Due to the accumulating evidence of the inverse association between aerobic fitness and stroke mortality, the third goal is to increase aerobic fitness. Patients entering physical rehabilitation programs should undergo preexercise evaluation to determine individual needs, limitations, and possible contraindications. The preexercise evaluation for stroke typically follows contemporary guidelines and includes a physical evaluation to identify neurological complications and other limiting medical conditions, and a graded exercise test if not contraindicated. Treadmill walking, arm ergometer, or leg ergometer protocols are often utilized for graded exercise testing in stroke patients depending on limitations. Results from preexercise evaluation are used to tailor exercise prescription to the individual needs of each patient.

Aerobic exercise programs for poststroke patients may include arm, leg, or arm and leg ergometer exercise 3 to 7 days a week for 20 to 60 minutes each session depending on level of fitness of patient with intensity tailored to patient needs. Intermittent sessions of 10 minutes each can be used if needed. Treadmill walking has the advantage of improving a task needed in everyday living. Resistance training including 10 to 15 repetitions with lower weight loads and utilizing all the major muscle groups in the body is recommended. Flexibility and neuromuscular training are also suggested so that range of motion and ADLs are improved (Chandler, 2014).

SUMMARY

Physical activity has major health benefits for individuals at any age. Remaining active throughout one's life span can reduce the risk for chronic diseases, reduce health care costs, and promote healthy aging. Exercise training that includes regimens of aerobic exercise, resistance training, and stretching can promote better fitness levels, maintain independent living, and further enhance health status and quality of life. Apparently healthy older adults beginning an exercise program for the first time, or planning to participate in a more vigorous program, should at least complete a self-administered preparticipation questionnaire. Individuals who have symptoms or diagnosed cardiovascular disease, pulmonary disease, or metabolic disease should get medical clearance before beginning an exercise program. Even persons with diagnosed health conditions and disease can benefit from exercise training. Following significant cardiac events or stroke, exercise is prescribed to reduce occurrence of future cardiac or stroke events, reduce risks, and improve functional capacity.

After reviewing this chapter, you should be able to:

- Discuss the most prevalent health problems in older adults (aged 65 and older).
- Identify the prevalent chronic diseases in older adults and the associated health care costs.
- Discuss the health risks of physical inactivity and the benefits of physical activity and exercise for the aging population.
- Define the terms related to health-related fitness and exercise training.
- Discuss preexercise screening, medical clearance, and exercise testing prior to starting an exercise program.
- Identify risks of exercise testing and exercise in general.
- Identify contraindications to exercise testing.
- Discuss supervised exercise programs for patients' postcardiac or stroke events.

REFERENCES

American College of Sports Medicine. (2014a). *ACSM's guidelines for exercise testing and prescription* (9th ed.). Baltimore, MD: Wolters Kluwer, Lippincott Williams & Wilkins.

American College of Sports Medicine. (2014b). *The basics of exercise training in seniors.* Retrieved from http://certification.acsm.org/blog/2014/january/the-basics-of-personal-training-for-seniors

American College of Sports Medicine. (2015). *Exercise and the older adult*. Retrieved from https://www.acsm.org/docs/current-comments/exerciseandtheolder adulCh

American Psychological Association. (2015). *Older adults' health and age-related changes*. Retrieved from https://www.apa.org/pi/aging/resources/guides/older.aspx

Centers for Disease Control and Prevention. (2015a). FastStats: Older person's health. Retrieved from www.cdc.gov/nchs/fastats/older-american-health.htm

Centers for Disease Control and Prevention. (2015b). *State-specific healthy life expectancy at age 65 years*. Retrieved from http://www.cdc.gov/mmwr/preview/mmwrhtml/mm6228a1.htm

Centers for Disease Control and Prevention. (2015c). *Target heart rate and estimated maximum heart rate*. Retrieved from http://www.cdc.gov/physicalactivity/basics/measuring/heartrate.htm

Centers for Disease Control and Prevention. (2015d). *Measuring physical activity intensity*. Retrieved from http://www.cdc.gov/physicalactivity/basics/measuring/index.html

Chandler, P. (2014). *Recovering from a stroke: The role of exercise*. Retrieved from http://dx.doi.org/10.1161/01.CIR.0000126280.65777.A4

Exercise Is Medicine. (2015). *Physical activity and NCDs*. Retrieved from www.exerciseismedicine.org/support_page.php?=3

Insel, P., & Roth, W. (2012). *Core concepts in health* (12th ed.). New York, NY: McGraw Hill.

National Heart, Lung, and Blood Institute. (2013). *What is cardiac rehabilitation?* Retrieved from http://www.nhlbi.nih.gov/health/health-topics/topics/rehab/

National Institute on Aging. (2014). *Exercise and physical activity: Your everyday guide from the National Institute on Aging*. Retrieved from https://www.nia.nih.gov/health/publication/exercise-physical-activity/introduction

Office of Disease Prevention and Health Promotion. (2015a). *Physical activity has many health benefits*. Retrieved from http://health.gov/paguidelines/guidelines/chapter2.aspx

Office of Disease Prevention and Health Promotion. (2015b). *Additional considerations for some adults*. Retrieved from http://health.gov/paguidelines/guidelines/chapter7.aspx

Ory, M., Resnick, M., Chodzko-Zajko, W., Buchner, D., & Bazzarre, T. (2005). *New ways of thinking about pre-activity screening for older adults. Medscape Pubic Health*. Retrieved from http://www.medscape.com/viewarticle/500790

President's Council on Fitness, Sports, and Nutrition. (2014). *Facts and statistics: Physical activity*. Retrieved from www.fitness.gov/resource-center/facts-and-statistics

Quinn, E. (2016). *What is VO2 Max in Athletic Training?* Retrieved from https://www.verywell.com/what-is-vo2-max-3120097

St. Onge, M., & Gallagher, D. (2010). Body composition changes with aging: The cause or the result of alterations in metabolic rate and macronutrient oxidation .*Nutrition, 26*(2), 152–155.

USA Triathlon. (2015). *Principles of exercise and sport training*. Retrieved from www.usatriathlon.org/about-multisport/mulitsort-zone/multisport-lab/articles/7-principlesoftraining-082812.aspx

World Health Organization. (2015). *Physical activity*. Retrieved from www.who.int/mediacentre/factsheets/fs385/en

CHAPTER 14

Policy Implications of Increasing Health Literacy Among Elders

RONALD A. HARRIS

This chapter discusses the policy implications of increasing health literacy among older adults. "Health literacy" may be defined as "the degree to which individuals have the capacity to obtain, process, and understand basic health information and services needed to make appropriate health decisions" (Parker, Ratzan, & Lurie, 2003). Generational differences distinguish older adults from the general population, including: education, socialization, and cognition. Research shows that older adults have limited functional health literacy and a lower quality of life (Hammad & Mulholland, 1992; Smith, et al., 2014). Low health literacy limits the ability of consumers to navigate the health system and obtain services (Bennett, Boyle, James, & Bennett, 2012; Boyle et al., 2013; Kobayashi, Wardle, Wolf, & Wagner, 2014). In a multicultural society, language acquisition is a barrier to health literacy (Yeo, 2009).

The target population for our focus on policies for health literacy is older adults. "Elders" refer to older adults among the general population aged 60 years and over for policy actions. This group is a socially constructed class identified by the government in the *Older Americans Act of 1965*. The aging network that was established by this federal program makes links across levels of government in the United States (Harris, 2012b). Life expectancy at birth for women was age 48 years in 1900. By 1965, average life expectancy had increased to 74 years and reached 81 years by 2013. As human longevity increased over the past century, the so-called "new-old" may not feel they belong to this class. They may reject the notion that older adults are a vulnerable subpopulation and require special policies.

Older adults who were educated before the innovation of medical technologies may not be aware of alternative treatments. They were socialized to rely upon agents, especially physicians, to make health care decisions without question. They may rely upon caregivers to make their decisions, because they are unable to make their own decisions due to cognitive impairments or physical incapacities from chronic diseases. Health literacy should increase their information to decide between alternative medical treatments. A consumer-driven approach to health care can improve market efficiency.

THE SOCIAL PROBLEM

As a society, the United States is not getting sufficient return on investment from spending on health care. We spend twice as much as most other developed countries on health care, but we rate way below them on health outcomes. Older adults account for most health care spending in our society, because we treat symptoms of the illnesses and are not so engaged in the prevention of disease. As much as three-quarters of the funds for health are spent on older adults, most of which is for end-of-life care. Policy alternatives are focused mostly on cost, and less on value for health care services (Garber, Goldman, & Jena, 2007).

The rising costs of health care have led policymakers to attempt to contain them. But such policies have limited impact in bending the cost curve downward, as medical technology often yields benefits over costs. Technological innovations in medicine are threatened by cost containment (Jessup, 2012; Rettig, 1994). Lopsided consumption of health care services across generations wherein older adults use most of the resources results in a wealth transfer from younger to older adults, especially for end-of-life care.

In Japan, an aging population has led to rising costs for health care, transferring social wealth from youth to elders. Despite a tradition of revering elders, Taro Aso, who is a Japanese finance minister, shared his sentiments about paying for end-of-life care. He recently said, "Let elderly people 'hurry up and die'" (McCurry, 2013). The Baby Boom generation began retiring in 2012. Eighty million people will retire over the next 20 years, increasing demands on health care and retirement systems in the United States.

THE AGENCY PROBLEM

In principal–agent relationships, like the doctor–patient relationship, the consumer (principal) incurs agency costs for monitoring the producer's (agent) performance, such as by acquiring information or obtaining a second medical opinion (Jensen & Meckling, 1976). The role of intermediaries in health care, such as insurers, and monopolization of information among health care providers is problematic for market efficiency. Another agency problem exists for the subpopulation of older adults who may be at least partly unable to make personal health care decisions and hence require help from caregivers.

Health care economics developed as a subfield because the market conditions are not conducive to efficiency. The basic assumptions of neoclassical economics are rational preferences, utility maximization, and complete information. When these basic conditions are obtained, the market will efficiently allocate resources in society, as if there is an invisible hand guiding all transactions. There is a gap in exchange between buyers and sellers, because of insurance. Insurers are the third-party payers and have stakes in exchange. When conditions for market competition are not met, the result is market failure. The four traditional market failures: public goods, externalities, natural monopolies, and information asymmetries are used to rationalize government policies (Weimer & Vining, 2015). Whenever governments intervene in markets, a reallocation of resources occurs that favors some special interests over others. Government failure can also result, sometimes through the unintended consequences of myopic health policies.

IMPERFECT INFORMATION

The problem is partly one of imperfect information needed to make an informed decision by consumers. Information is not free to produce or consume, except for any positive externalities that might follow as byproducts of production allowing free riders. Arrow (1963) said that when there is uncertainty, accurate information or knowledge becomes a valuable commodity. "Information, in the form of skilled care, is precisely what is being bought from most physicians" (p. 946). Therefore, medical markets are actually markets for information. "Diagnostic and treatment information are extremely valuable to patients faced with decisions about what health care services to consume" (Haas-Wilson, 2001). Now in the information age, consumers have multiple sources of information that are independent from their physicians. There has been an explosive growth in the amount of health care information available online. Most likely even the most well-informed consumers will continue to follow their physicians' medical advice.

SUPPLIER-INDUCED DEMAND

Asymmetric information where sellers have superior knowledge about services and products leads to an unfavorable bargaining position for consumers. In health care markets, consumer sovereignty is in jeopardy, because of "supplier-induced demand." Physicians with superior information can induce their information-poor patients to spend more on unnecessary medical treatments (Wennberg, Barnes, & Zubkoff, 1982). Cutler, Skinner, Stern, and Wennberg (2013) studied health care expenditures to determine whether patient demand-side factors or physician supply-side factors can explain regional variation in Medicare spending. They found that patient demand does not explain variations in health care expenditures. More importantly, physician beliefs about treatment were the single most important factor for explaining variations: "36% of end-of-life spending and 17% of U.S. health care spending are associated with physician beliefs unsupported by clinical evidence."

CONSUMER SOVEREIGNTY

When consumers acquire better information to make health care decisions, they are able to correct agency problems, such as supplier-induced demand by physicians. This could lead to increased consumption of health care services, but certainly shifts power towards them and away from suppliers. However, pharmaceutical costs could continue to increase as consumers demand prescriptions for brand name drugs from physicians in response to direct-to-consumer advertising, which is also health literacy.

Payers (agents) intervene on behalf of consumers through payment mechanisms and gatekeepers to reduce such costs. They offer health information to consumers directly, which can guide them to appropriate providers. This increases consumer satisfaction.

Just as basic K–12 education creates the highest level of human development among nations, basic literacy in health should also generate the highest level of health. Elders with lower educational levels compared with subsequent generations and who may tend to trust their physicians more, might rely more on medical advice than younger patients.

HEALTH POLICY

There are many health policies in place to address health literacy in our society. "Health policy refers to decisions, plans, and actions that are undertaken to achieve specific health care goals within a society"

(World Health Organization, 2015). Policies are made by producers, payers, and consumers. The payers, especially governments, are intermediaries between the producers and consumers. Private payers, like health insurance companies, make their own policies, but are also regulated by governments. Governments respond to demand for health policies from private payers, producers, and consumers. Health care is highly regulated in the United States and developed nations.

People who survive acute disease and injuries will succumb to chronic disease, inevitably. Prevention is preferred to treatment, not only because it can lower long-term health care costs, but also because it can prolong life with higher quality of experience. Fries (2005) has proposed compressing morbidity to improve the quality of life for older adults and shorten the time frame in the life cycle when expensive treatments often occur for end-of-life care. Fries (2005) recommended these changes to our health policy:

1. There should be no mandatory retirement age.
2. Creative vocational opportunities should be available.
3. Health enhancement programs must begin early in adult life.
4. We should seek deinstitutionalization of long-term care programs.
5. Programs should stimulate the independence of individuals.
6. We need to look closely at how our laws and our customs may affect the independent expression of vitality in the older individual.

We could change our social and health policies to implement recommendations to compress morbidity in the following ways. Retirement could become optional with a means test for those who can afford it, while disability pensions could readily substitute for extant retirement plans. Continuing education programs for second and third careers should be established for elders. Education for the prevention of chronic disease should be essential to prepare younger adults for a future as elders. Support for aging-in-place programs that allow older adults to stay within their communities should be provided (Harris, 2012a). Rather than view older adults as experiencing their second childhood, they should get respect for living long enough to acquire wisdom that could be imparted to the young.

STAKEHOLDER ANALYSIS

Key stakeholders for health literacy include: producers, payers, and consumers who influence decision-making processes for health policy (Brugha & Varvasovszky, 2000). The producers are the hospitals, clinicians, and vendors. The clinicians include physicians, nurses, and specialty providers. Vendors include information technology, the pharmaceutical industry, medical device manufacturers, and suppliers. The payers are employers, governments, and private individuals. The consumers include employees, recipients of government insurance, such as Tri-Care, Medicare, Medicaid, and S-CHIP. The self-employed pay for their health insurance and the underemployed get subsidies.

Each stakeholder provides or acquires information about health care services to improve their market position. Producers historically monopolized health information, which is being widely disseminated today through other channels, like online portals. Payers want to inform consumers to help them make better choices and improve their outcomes, which helps to reduce costs and increase efficient allocation of resources. Consumers seek information to obtain better health care services for improved quality.

Health care provision is an industry comprising at least one-sixth of the U.S. economy and should grow to one-fifth soon. At the federal policy level, there is a National Action Plan to Improve Health Literacy (Koh, 2010). The national plan has seven goals:

1. Develop and disseminate health and safety information that is accurate, accessible, and actionable.
2. Promote changes in the health care delivery system that improve information, communication, informed decision making, and access to health services.
3. Incorporate accurate and standards-based health and developmentally appropriate health and science information and curricula into child care and education through the university level.
4. Support and expand local efforts to provide adult education, English-language instruction, and culturally and linguistically appropriate health information services in the community.
5. Build partnerships, develop guidance, and change policies.
6. Increase basic research and the development, implementation, and evaluation of practices and interventions to improve health literacy.
7. Increase the dissemination and use of evidence-based health literacy practices and interventions.

The purpose of the national plan is to educate the public, especially prospective patients, about health to prevent the overuse and misuse of scarce medical resources. According to Koh and colleagues (2012), the National Action Plan to Improve Health Literacy, the Plain Writing Act of 2010, and the Affordable Care Act (ACA) of 2010, make literacy a priority.

THE AFFORDABLE CARE ACT

Policy makers in the United States have changed the focus from treatment to prevention in health care with the Affordable Care Act of 2010 and utilized additional strategies to improve health literacy. Title V of the ACA defines "health literacy" as "the degree to which an individual has the capacity to obtain, communicate, process, and understand basic health information and services to make appropriate health decisions." But critics of the ACA claim that Americans with low health literacy will benefit the least from the policy (Somers & Mahadevan, 2010). Nearly 36% of America's adult population, which is about 87 million adults in the United States, are functionally illiterate (Vernon, Trujillo, Rosenbaum, & DeBuono, 2007).

PATIENT EDUCATION

Older adults can improve their health literacy by participating in patient educational programs, such as the Chronic Disease Self-Management Program (CDSMP) designed by Lorig (1996). Teaching self-management skills to older adults has proven more effective in improving clinical outcomes than providing information without any teaching activities (Bodenheimer Lorig, Holman, & Grumbach, 2002). Subjects covered in CDSMP workshops include:

1. Techniques to deal with problems such as frustration, fatigue, pain, and isolation
2. Appropriate exercise for maintaining and improving strength, flexibility, and endurance
3. Appropriate use of medications
4. Communicating effectively with family, friends, and health professionals
5. Nutrition
6. Decision making
7. How to evaluate new treatments

CDSMP patient education was delivered to more than 500 participants at Senior Centers in Louisiana, from 2010 to 2012 (Harris, Kopera-Frye, Estrade, & Hicks, 2013). More than 75% of them completed the 6-week program. Among the statistically significant findings was a reduction in health care utilization, including emergency room visits and hospitalizations. This program should reduce costs for delivery of health care services and also improve health literacy among participants, who can live longer and enjoy a higher quality of life.

POLICY IMPLICATIONS

What are the policy implications of low health literacy among elders? The inefficiencies resulting from information asymmetry are costly for health care and the society. Vernon and colleagues (2007) find that "$106–$238 billion is lost every year on health care costs due to a disconnect in the delivery of health information and communication methods of health care providers and the ability of adults to obtain, process, and understand health information." Direct medical costs for chronic conditions were $510 billion in 2000 and are expected to double to $1 trillion by 2020 (Parker et al., 2003).

What are the policy implications of increasing health literacy among elders? A disruptive technology like the Internet provides new sources of information to patients. Modern consumers of health care services can use mobile phone health applications (Broderick et al., 2014). Information is power for producers, payers, and consumers alike, but we can also experience information overload. Patient educational programs like CDSMP focus on what is important in health. Imperfect information could make people feel powerless to act on their health needs and interact with the health care system.

CONCLUSIONS

We can save health dollars in treatment costs by educating older adults to make better choices to prevent or to self-manage chronic diseases. Emergency medical care is quite expensive and often results from failure to manage chronic conditions or prevent them. Because older adults often have many chronic diseases, prevention should target younger people and patient education about self-management should target the elderly.

By increasing health literacy in older adults, consumers should be able to make more informed decisions about illness prevention and health care treatments. Because older adults usually have one or more chronic illnesses, an increase in their managerial capacity to engage with the health system should reduce costs of emergency treatment. Consumers who can acquire relevant health information should be expected to make better preventive decisions and require less emergency treatment. The main problem of health care markets has been intermediaries, such as insurers, involved in consumption, which affects resource allocation in ways not expected in idealized competitive markets.

Should we remake society following the recommendations of Fries (2005) to compress morbidity in the life cycle, our health policy will change quite dramatically. It would mean ending retirement, changing career paths as we move though the life cycle, aging-in-place instead of long-term care facilities, and recovering dignity for older adults through rules. Since we have a hodge-podge of stakeholders with competing interests over provision of health care, attempts were made to establish policy goals by the federal government, such as the ACA. But the ACA hardly addresses low health literacy, which is seen as the responsibility of health professionals, rather than patients.

REFERENCES

Affordable Care Act. (2010). 42 U.S.C. § 18001.

Arrow, K. J. (1963). Uncertainty and the welfare economics of medical care. *American Economic Review, 53*(5), 941–973.

Bennett, J. S., Boyle, P. A., James, B. D., & Bennett, D. A. (2012). Correlates of health and financial literacy in older adults without dementia. *BioMed Central Geriatrics, 12*, 30.

Bodenheimer, T., Lorig, K., Holman, H., & Grumbach, K. (2002). Patient self-management of chronic disease in primary care. *Journal of the American Medical Association, 288*(19), 2469–2475.

Boyle, P. A., Yu, L., Wilson, R. S., Segawa, E., Buchman, A. S., & Bennett, D. A. (2013). Cognitive decline impairs financial and health literacy among community-based older persons without dementia. *Psychology and Aging, 28*(3), 614–624.

Broderick, J., Devine, T., Langhans, E., Lemerise, A. J., Lier, S., & Harris, L. (2014, January 28). *Designing health literate mobile apps*. Institute of Medicine. National Academy of Sciences. http://health.gov/communication/literacy/BPH-HealthLiterateApps.pdf

Brugha, R., & Varvasovszky, Z. (2000). Stakeholder analysis: A review. *Health Policy and Planning, 15*(3), 239–246.

Cutler, D., Skinner, J., Stern, A. D., & Wennberg, D. (2013, August). *Physician beliefs and patient preferences: A new look at regional variation in health care spending*. Working Paper 19320. Cambridge, MA: National Bureau of Economic Research.

Fries, J. F. (2005). The compression of morbidity. *Milbank Quarterly, 83*(4), 801–823. doi:10.1111/j.1468-0009.2005.00401.x

Garber, A., Goldman, D. P., & Jena, A. B. (2007). The promise of healthcare cost containment. *Health Affairs, 26*(6), 1545–1547.

Haas-Wilson, D. (2001). Arrow and the information market failure in health care: The changing content and sources of health care information. *Journal of Health Politics, Policy and Law, 26*(5), 1031–1044.

Hammad, A. E., & Mulholland, C. (1992). Functional literacy, health, and quality of life. *Annals of the American Academy of Political and Social Science, 520*, 103–120.

Harris, R. A. (2012a). Louisiana answers for living at home: State pilot program for aging in place. *International Journal of Aging and Society, 1*(1), 51–64.

Harris, R. A. (2012b). The Louisiana aging network: Analyzing an organizational network. *International Journal of Health, Wellness and Society, 1*(4), 19–32.

Harris, R. A., Kopera-Frye, K., Estrade, M. W., & Hicks, W. J. (2013). Your life, your health! Chronic disease self-management education in Louisiana. *International Journal of Health, Wellness and Society, 3*(2), 1–12.

Jensen, M. C., & Meckling, W. H. (1976). Theory of the firm: Managerial behavior, agency costs and ownership structure. *Journal of Financial Economics, 3*(4), 305–360.

Jessup, A. (2012). *Health care cost containment and medical innovation.* U.S. Department of Health and Human Services. Retrieved from https://aspe.hhs.gov/basic-report/health-care-cost-containment-and-medical-innovation

Kobayashi, L. C., Wardle, J., Wolf, M. S., & Wagner, C. (2014). Aging and functional health literacy: A systematic review and meta-analysis. *Journal of Gerontology, 71,* 445–457.

Koh, H. K. (2010). *National action plan to improve health literacy.* Washington, DC: U.S. Department of Health and Human Services. http://health.gov/communication/hlactionplan/pdf/Health_Literacy_Action_Plan.pdf

Koh, H. K., Berwick, D. M., Clancy, C. M., Baur, C., Brach, C., Harris, L. M., & Zerhsen, E. G. (2012). New federal policy initiatives to boost health literacy can help the nation move beyond the cycle of costly "crisis care." *Health Affairs, 31*(2), 434–443.

Lorig, K. (1996). Chronic disease self-management: A model for tertiary prevention. *American Behavioral Science, 39,* 767–783.

McCurry, J. (2013, January 22). Let elderly people "hurry up and die", says Japanese minister. *Guardian.* Retrieved from http://www.theguardian.com/world/2013/jan/22/elderly-hurry-up-die-japanese

Older Americans Act of 1965. (1965). 79 Stat. 218.

Parker, R. M., Ratzan, S. C., & Lurie, N. (2003). Health literacy: A policy challenge for advancing high-quality health care. *Health Affairs, 22*(4), 147–153.

Rettig, R. A. (1994). Medical innovation duels cost containment. *Health Affairs, 13*(3), 7–27.

Smith, S. G., O'Conor, R., Curtis, L. M., Waite, K., Deary, I. J., Paasche-Orlow, M., & Wolf, M. S. (2014). Low health literacy predicts decline in physical function among older adults: Findings from the LitCog cohort study. *Journal of Epidemiology and Community Health, 69*(5), 474–480.

Somers, S. A., & Mahadevan, R. (2010, November). *Health literacy implications of the Affordable Care Act.* Washington, DC: Center for Health Care Strategies. http://www.chcs.org/media/Health_Literacy_Implications_of_the_Affordable_Care_Act.pdf

Vernon, J. A., Trujillo, A., Rosenbaum, S., & DeBuono, B. (2007). *Low health literacy: Implications for national health policy.* Washington, DC: The George Washington University.

Weimer, D. L., & Vining, A. R. (2011). *Policy analysis* (5th ed.). New York, NY: Longman.

Wennberg, J. E., Barnes, B. A., & Zubkoff, M. (1982). Professional uncertainty and the problem of supplier-induced demand. *Social Science and Medicine, 16,* 811–823.

World Health Organization. (2015). Health policy. Retrieved from http://www.who.int/topics/health-policy/en

Yeo, G. (2009). How will the U.S. healthcare system meet the challenge of the ethno geriatric imperative? *Journal of the American Geriatrics Society, 57*(7), 1278–1285.

CHAPTER 15

Where Do We Go From Here With Health Literacy?

R. V. RIKARD AND JULIE MCKINNEY

The purpose of our chapter is to provide some direction on where do we go from here with health literacy. At first, we thought the task of providing directions would be relatively easy given the volumes of research on health literacy in general, and specifically health literacy among older adults. However, we realized that we could not simply summarize all the research focusing on older adults and health literacy. Therefore, we begin with a broad look at the field of health literacy and a working conceptual framework of health literacy. Next, we highlight theories from the fields of adult learning and educational and social gerontology that may guide future health literacy practice and research with older adults. We then discuss the state of health literacy measures and advancements in measurement. We turn our attention to point out a new direction and focus on health literacy among older adults. We conclude the chapter with a summary, and encourage readers to consider the following question: Where do you want to go from here with health literacy?

HISTORY, DEFINITION AND CONCEPTUAL FRAMEWORK

"Health literacy" is an unwieldy concept. The challenge of defining it was once described to us as being like "wrestling worms." Identifying and defining the concept of health literacy is difficult because health literacy encompasses so many other concepts, disciplines, and fields of study. For example, how do we distinguish it from health education, health communication, plain language, or cultural competency? To understand where to go from here with health literacy, we begin with a brief background.

Health literacy has been an evolving concept for about 20 years, since people in the health and literacy worlds first began to notice the

249

connection between the two fields. This began with an awareness of the challenges faced by people with limited literacy skills in accessing health information and care. This awareness was catalyzed by the realization that a shocking proportion of American adults had limited literacy skills. The U.S. Department of Education completed its first national survey of adult literacy skills in 1993, and found that more than half of the adults had skills that were limited enough to affect their ability to engage in many of the benefits of society (Kirsch, 1993). These benefits, of course, include engaging effectively with health information and services. Thus, the early concept of health literacy was that it referred to a set of skills that people have or lack that help them to read health-related written information. Consequently, early definitions of health literacy were focused on the reading abilities of individuals (Figure 15.1).

This new epiphany about the nation's literacy challenges led to a closer look at written health information, which revealed a staggering mismatch between the average person's ability to read and understand health information and the level of difficulty of the information being given to them by health care providers and educators. On average, health care materials were written at a college level, while the average reading level of adults was about eighth grade (Dowe, Lawrence, Carlson, & Keyserling, 1997; Rudd, Anderson, Oppenheimer, & Nath, 2007).

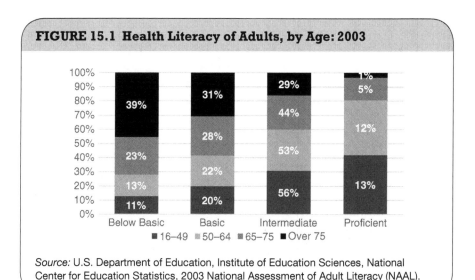

FIGURE 15.1 Health Literacy of Adults, by Age: 2003

Source: U.S. Department of Education, Institute of Education Sciences, National Center for Education Statistics, 2003 National Assessment of Adult Literacy (NAAL).

This, of course, has important relevance for the field of gerontology. As expected, these literacy challenges were magnified as one's age increased. Seniors' literacy skills were confirmed to be significantly lower than younger adults, even after controlling for other confounding factors. The reasons for this include cognitive decline, isolation, and less ongoing use of one's literacy skills in everyday life (Kirsch, 1993). Later, when measures of *health literacy* were introduced, the same trend persisted (Baker, Gazmararian, Sudano, & Patterson, 2000; Kutner, Greenburg, Jin, & Paulsen, 2006).

Now that there was an awareness of Americans' poor literacy skills, and an understanding of its implications for health, the concept of "health literacy skills" gained momentum. New screening tests were developed to screen patients' health literacy skills so that they could be compared with the demand that was required of them in health care settings. These first tests included the Rapid Estimate of Adults Literacy in Medicine (REALM) and the Test of Functional Health Literacy Assessment (TOFHLA). They were not founded on any specific definition, and were limited to simple, text-based tasks like recognizing a health-related word and filling in a blank word in a sentence. Later in the chapter we discuss how these screening and measurement tools have changed over time.

The second national survey of adult literacy completed in 2003 included a section to test specifically for health literacy skills. There were 28 items on the survey that asked respondents to answer questions based on typical health-information materials that included text and numerical charts. The results confirmed that over half the adult population have marginal health-literacy skills. The sound bite from this survey was that over 90 million adults in the United States have trouble understanding and acting on health information (Nielsen-Bohlman, Panzer, & Kindig, 2004). This galvanized the medical world, in large part due to a report from the Institute of Medicine (IOM), *Health Literacy: A Prescription to End Confusion*. This report used the following definition of health literacy: "the degree to which individuals have the capacity to obtain, process, and understand basic health information and services needed to make appropriate health decisions" (Nielsen-Bohlman et al., 2004; Ratzan & Parker, 2000). While this sound bite cited over half the population as being at risk, a second look at the National Assessment of Adult Literacy (NAAL) data revealed that actually only 12% of American adults have *proficient* health literacy skills. And for adults over the age of 65, only 3% had proficient health literacy skill (Pleasant, 2008). Proficient skills are the level that is needed to adequately take care of one's health, especially with the complex medical needs that older adults routinely face.

The report was widely cited and used by medical researchers and practitioners and the IOM definition came to be the most commonly used one. The definition expands on earlier definitions by adding the elements of *finding* and the ability to *understand* information. However, this definition of health literacy continued to focus on a set of skills that individuals either possess or lack. The "blame-the-patient" approach was a limited way to conceptualize the problem of low health literacy. While the definition did not acknowledge the skills and abilities of providers, the IOM report did discuss the role of providers in addressing the problem and led to a growing understanding that health care providers and systems present barriers to care and should share the responsibility for improving the situation.

The new concept of health literacy as a shared burden took off and created widespread efforts to train health care providers on how to communicate more effectively with their patients who had low literacy skills. However, few definitions acknowledged the importance of the provider. One of the first definitions that directly addressed skills of the providers was that from the *Calgary Charter on Health Literacy: Rationale and Core Principles for the Development of Health Literacy Curricula*, as shown in Box 15.1 (Coleman et al., 2009).

The conceptualization was important in the evolution of health literacy in a few ways. First, the Calgary Charter definition clearly acknowledged that health literacy is a two-way street: It includes skills and abilities that apply to providers and systems, not just individuals. The Calgary Charter's core principles focused on efforts to train providers and implement systems change as a method for improving health

---

BOX 15.1 Health Literacy Defined

- Health literacy allows the public and personnel working in all health-related contexts to find, understand, evaluate, communicate, and use information.
- Health literacy is the use of a wide range of skills that improve the ability of people to act on information in order to live healthier lives.
- These skills include reading, writing, listening, speaking, numeracy, and critical analysis, as well as communication and interaction skills.

literacy and thus health outcomes. The Charter also encouraged the field to develop ways to measure the health literacy of the providers and systems, not just the patients. However, today there are still few measures focused on provider and system health literacy.

Second, the Calgary Charter definition broke down health literacy into a series of five discreet abilities: To find, understand, evaluate, communicate, and use health information. In order to have a high level of health literacy, an individual needs to be able to accomplish the five abilities; and a system or provider needs to enable their clients to easily accomplish the five abilities. This provides a very specific framework of what to measure, and also allows the development of educational programs and other interventions that specifically address these five abilities.

Third, the Calgary Charter concept encourages a focus that goes beyond reading and understanding health information to explore how people *use* the information to make changes that improve health. It can be seen as a theory of behavioral change and built into a logic model for implementing change (Pleasant, 2014). This is an operational definition that has the potential to allow us to measure health literacy (through the five components) and to develop interventions that can be tailored to specific settings, health conditions, or audiences. Using these five components as the framework for measuring the construct, we should be able to compare the results across these settings. In other words, if we were to compare the health literacy levels of diabetic patients in a neighborhood clinic to those of chronic obstructive pulmonary disease (COPD) patients or nursing home residents, we could do this by measuring their ability to find information, understand it, evaluate it, communicate about it, and use it in the context of their disease and setting.

THEORY

The majority of health literacy research is atheoretical, and health literacy research that is theoretically driven *and* focuses on older adults is nearly nonexistent (see Smith & Hudson, 2012 for an exception). A theory is a statement or explanation of how and why two or more concepts should be related. More importantly, theories provide a framework to guide and understand the meaning of research and the development of programs and interventions. The lack of theoretically driven research means that practitioners and researchers cannot explain the consistent research finding of lower health literacy among older adults. In other words, what are the full ranges of factors that account for the decline in health literacy levels among older adults? We highlight below some theories from the fields of Adult Learning and Social Gerontology that may guide future health literacy practice and research with older adults.

ADULT LEARNING

Good health depends on actions that we take after learning what we need to do and how to do it. It also depends on how prepared we are to take those actions with initiative and confidence. So in order to promote health, people must not only learn information and skills, but also incorporate those skills into their daily habits with the intent of improving their lives. Since the field of adult education is built on principles of using new skills to improve one's station in life, the theoretical frameworks from this field can be useful when looking at health literacy. We will look at three: andragogy, transformational learning, and critical learning.

Knowles (1973) introduced the concept of "andragogy," which distinguished the process by which adults learn as opposed to children. This included the ideas that adults must be self-directed in their learning and draw upon their experiences in order to make sense of new information and skills. Adults also use a problem-centered approach: What they learn should be used to fix a certain problem in their lives; and they need to know *why* they need to know something new (Knowles, 1973, 1992). Auerbach's focus on participatory education as an essential component is also a key ingredient in approaching health education (Auerbach, 1992). When adults are involved in doing something in the context of learning new skills and information, they are more likely to use that information in their lives. We can see how these theories could inform health education and health literacy strategies.

Transformational learning is that which brings about a shift in how people see themselves in relation to the community or world around them. This requires a trusting environment and a good understanding of one's learners. If you see the target population of health promotion efforts as the "learners," you can see how this approach would help to encourage health care providers and systems to "know their audience" in a way that improves these efforts. But this can be taken a step further.

The teachings of Paulo Freire bring transformational learning to a new focus of questioning one's present position. Freire's theory of critical learning aims to equalize the power dynamic between the "teacher" and the "learner." This theory asserts that the relationship between the teacher and learner is equal, and that they work together to incorporate new ideas into the lives of the individuals and the community as a whole. The process involves a highly engaged problem-solving approach, and the ultimate goal is to transform the status of the individual and community in political, social, and economic arenas (Freire, 1970). This concept could help to create a better model for the patient–provider relationship and for the process by which decisions are made about care, treatment, and behavioral change. Our current health care culture is quite hierarchical and features a significant power dynamic between health care providers and patients. Studies have shown that patients' blood pressures actually rises when a "white-coat" walks into the room (Franklin, Thijs, Hansen, O'Brien, & Staessen, 2013). So the critical learning theory has some useful elements that could help to create a more balanced power dynamic and help empower community members—especially ones like older adults who are already marginalized—in being more engaged in their own health care.

SOCIAL GERONTOLOGY

The stress process is the most prevalent social framework to examine the aspects of aging and health. Pearlin (1989) emphasized that life changes are not necessarily negative and that life-course transitions are not necessarily associated with decreased psychological well-being. Pearlin (1989) theorized that transitions in the life course lead to changes in social and economic conditions that may pose "life strains." In terms of older adults, level of health literacy may either increase or decrease the impact of stress. Thus, higher levels of health literacy may buffer the "life strains" of aging.

The health outcomes that are a result of cumulative inequality are observed in later life. Cumulative inequalities are an important theoretical development to understanding the overall impact of social inequality on health outcomes among older adults. However, few studies demonstrate linkages between early life conditions to late life outcomes. As a theoretical perspective to examine health literacy among older adults, cumulative inequality requires understanding the factors that shape an older adult's level of health knowledge and action. Therefore, a life-course perspective is also needed to examine the extent of life events.

A life-course perspective examines the life events that shift and change health outcomes with advancing age. The concept of "linked lives" is the most useful tool to examine and understand the actions and interactions of family members over time. To understand both expected and unexpected life-course events, there is a need to appreciate events that occur over time. Therefore, not only is the impact of life events important but also the way in which people experience, adapt, and find social support to cope with life events. Employing the life-course perspective highlights that health literacy changes over time. Moreover, examining health literacy as a trait that changes and the importance of social support suggests that health literacy is more than simply an individual deficit. Instead, health literacy is social and malleable. This opens the door to exploring how we can best improve health literacy over time as a route to better health in later life.

HEALTH LITERACY MEASUREMENT

As with any relatively new field, the tools for measuring health literacy are still in a fairly early stage of development. In addition, effective methods to measure health literacy as a multifaceted concept are challenging to create. Furthermore, since a theoretical concept and widely accepted definition have yet to be agreed upon in the field, it has proved impossible to create measurement tools that reflect the theory and definition of health literacy.

The first health literacy measurement tools, as we mentioned earlier, were simple screeners to test individual health literacy. These were very rudimentary, and limited to assessing simple reading tasks. The REALM asked respondents to read and pronounce a list of health and medical words. The TOFHLA was a set of cloze exercises where a person had to fill in the blank in a sentence. At the time, these were being used to test the health literacy of patients in a clinical setting and needed to be brief and easy to administer. Now that the field is moving toward testing more complex aspects of health literacy, the tools are evolving, yet are still hampered by the lack of a theoretical foundation.

In 2010, there was an attempt to survey the field and reach some consensus about the state of health literacy measurements (Pleasant & McKinney, 2011). One of the most comprehensive groups of health literacy professionals is an online forum called the Health Literacy Discussion List (HLDL), which reaches over 1,500 diverse professionals from around the world with an interest in health literacy. At the time, the HLDL was administered by a division of the U.S. Department of Education, the Literacy Information and Communication System (LINCS), although it is now supported by the Institute for Healthcare Advancement (IHA). There was a rich discussion with the list members about health literacy measurement and over 100 members answered a survey to determine the field's opinions about what a health literacy concept should include and what features a measurement tool should have. There was general consensus that health literacy went beyond reading ability, that it is a determinant of health status, and that its effects extend beyond the clinical setting into many other domains of society. There was also consensus that a measurement tool should include these skills as they relate to health information: finding it, understanding it, evaluating or processing it, communicating about it, and using it to make informed choices about health (Pleasant & McKinney, 2011).

A second discussion revealed that a new approach to measuring health literacy was needed, one that was based on a theoretical foundation, treated health literacy as a latent concept, and captured the whole set of skills agreed on in the earlier survey. Two other key components deemed important were that new measures allow us to (a) measure health literacy of both individuals *and* providers and systems; and (b) make comparisons across contexts such as population, condition, and setting (Pleasant, McKinney, & Rikard, 2011).

Despite progress in the number and scope of new measures, there remain limitations. There are now over 50 measures of individual health literacy that have been developed for various populations (Haun, Valerio, McCormack, Sørensen, & Paasche-Orlow, 2014). However, each measure does not evaluate the same aspects of health literacy since the measures were developed independently of each other and without a cohesive foundation. Therefore, the measures cannot be used to compare across studies and populations.

Methodologically, the TOFHLA and REALM represent a first generation of health literacy assessment tools developed using Classical Test Theory. Keep in mind that first generation health literacy measures cannot be used to compare across studies and populations. An emerging second generation of assessment tools are based on strong psychometric properties and include: items from the NAAL (Baldi et al., 2009), the Health Literacy Skills Instrument (HLSI; McCormack et al., 2010), the Mandarian Health Literacy Scale (MHLS; Tsai, Lee, Tsai, & Kuo, 2011), and the Health Literacy Questionnaire (Osborne, Batterham, Elsworth, Hawkins, & Buchbinder, 2013).

There is some progress in assessing the skills of the provider and system side of the equation. There are new approaches to measuring what is called "organizational health literacy" (OHL). These involve getting information from providers, administrators, and ideally patients and assessing how well the organization operates in accordance with health literacy principles. In 2012 the Institute of Medicine developed a set of

10 attributes that a health care organization should have in order to be considered health literate (Brach et al., 2012). These attributes provided a framework for creating a new series of measurement tools and have also formed the basis of intervention efforts. However, there are few measures of how well providers themselves communicate in a health literate way and lower barriers to patient understanding. There are ongoing efforts to prioritize the competencies that should be considered essential for medical and health professionals (Coleman, Hudson, & Maine, 2013).

Finally, there have yet to be measures of public health literacy or community health literacy. These would presumably assess how well groups of individuals and systems work together to create an environment where it is easy for the public to find health information that they can understand, evaluate, communicate about, and use to take action for improving their health. This would be especially useful for a community of older adults, who have specialized strengths, needs, and challenges that relate to information, communication, and health.

FROM DESCRIPTION TO INTERVENTION

Despite the limitations of the existing tools to measure health literacy, there is a sizable evidence base for some important aspects. The aspects include the mismatch between skills and demand, the prevalence of poor health literacy in various subpopulations and clinical settings, and the strong association between low health literacy and poor health outcomes. At this point, we can be confident of the descriptive aspects of individuals' health literacy and the impact of low health literacy. We must point our efforts in a new direction. For example, there is now a need to study the health literacy of providers and systems, community and public health literacy, and the effectiveness of different solutions particularly with the growth of the aging population.

What We Already Know

As mentioned earlier, we have much evidence to back up the mismatch between health literacy skills of individuals and the literacy demand of health-related forms, instructions, and educational information that is available. So we know that people are too often faced with information that is above their ability to read, understand, and make use of. The mismatch is exacerbated for seniors who have even lower health literacy skills yet ever greater need for them. There are ongoing efforts to create information that is more appropriate for people with lower literacy and health literacy skills. The plain language movement has created a wealth of support for making written information easier to understand. There are now guidelines, policies, training materials, and standards that support materials developers in creating materials that are easier to understand and more actionable. In other words, fewer people will take one look and throw the materials in the trash; conversely, more people will read, understand, and take action.

We also have plenty of evidence to show that low health literacy is widespread in the United States, particularly among older adults. According to the NAAL, only 12% of American adults have proficient health literacy levels (Nielsen-Bohlman et al., 2004). Many other studies reveal poor health literacy skills in more specific settings and populations. While we know that poor health literacy affects people of all backgrounds, educational levels, and socioeconomic groups, we also know that certain groups have significantly lower levels, and this leads to health disparities. The elderly (Rootman & Ronson, 2005; Sudore et al., 2006), minorities, people from low socioeconomic backgrounds, and people who have not completed high school have disproportionally lower health literacy levels, and ultimately poorer health outcomes.

Research from study after study supports the finding that both literacy and specifically health literacy affect health outcomes. People with lower literacy skills or lower health literacy levels are consistently more likely to have worse health outcomes (Baker et al., 2000; Kutner et al., 2006; Rudd et al., 2007). Many of the reasons for the association are well documented. Low health literacy leads to misuse of medication, poor control of chronic conditions, increased risk of hospitalization (Baker et al., 2002), increased health care visits (Sanders, Thompson, & Wilkinson, 2007), and decreased knowledge of chronic health conditions (Williams, Baker, Parker, & Nurss, 1998). Health literacy of health care clients in a variety of clinical settings has been measured and shown to affect their respective treatments and outcomes. Furthermore, when other factors are taken into account, such as age, ethnicity, educational background, and socioeconomic status (SES), health literacy is a stronger predictor of poor health outcomes.

What We Need to Know

There is excellent descriptive data about the prevalence of low health literacy and health outcomes. The field of health literacy is ready to move into a new era of exploration. Research can now focus on the health literacy of providers and systems and the effectiveness of different solutions and interventions. There is also interest in branching out from studying clinical encounters and looking more closely at a broader view that includes community and public health literacy.

Exploring the Skills of Providers and Systems

There is growing acceptance of the two-way-street view of health literacy: Health outcomes depend not only on the skills of the individual, but also on the skills of the provider. In addition, the number of barriers in the health care system limits patients' ability to understand important information and take actions that will improve their health. In fact, there is now a comprehensive set of resources that help providers to communicate better with patients, or guide hospitals in lowering the health literacy-related barriers to care. This is a trend that should continue and develop.

Testing the Effectiveness of Solutions and Interventions

There is also, as we have discussed, some measures of OHL. These measures have been used mostly to help individual health care organizations determine which attributes to focus on in order to lower their health literacy barriers and improve care. However, such an approach is a shot in the dark to inform what kind of overall interventions are important for a health care organization. New OHL research should focus on assessing organizations before and after different interventions. The new research will ideally include longitudinal study designs to capture how interventions contribute to improved health literacy. The findings will provide the field of health literacy with evidence-based best practices and documented return on investment (ROI) outcomes. These ROI outcomes are especially important because they will show the worth of health literacy interventions to health system administrators, whose support is essential in order to fund and implement these intervention strategies.

The same research agenda is true to assess individual-level health literacy interventions. With all the research that has been done to determine the dismal level of health literacy, very little has been studied as to how best to improve health literacy in the general population, let alone certain subsets such as older adults. Some studies have revealed that teaching health literacy in the context of adult education classes can improve individuals' skills, self-efficacy, and intentions to act. Some behavioral changes have also been noted, such as getting flu shots or screening tests. Yet, there has not been enough to compare different educational approaches and provide evidence to determine the best practices. There are also different populations to consider, of course. The best approach to teach new immigrants who are learning English will be different from teaching seniors.

Social Support and Engagement

New research is needed to explore what other aspects of social or relational support can contribute to improving health literacy and ultimately lead to better health among older adults. Often those who struggle most with the effects of low health literacy also have poor social support networks, minimal civic participation, limited employment, and little access to health information. Older adults are more likely than other age groups to experience the challenge of declining social support, which has been shown to be a factor in living a healthier life to an advanced age (Perls, Bochen, Freeman, Alpert, & Silver, 1999). Therefore, focusing on a range of social aspects that may contribute to a person's level of health literacy will inform new interventions that could help older adults live a healthier life.

CONCLUSION

Years ago, what started as a vague connection between literacy skills and health grew into a new field of research and practice, now widely recognized as health literacy. Early research succeeded in describing the issue in good detail. We learned that a huge proportion of adults have limited ability to navigate the maze of information that is meant to help them stay healthy, and we also know that this limited ability leads to poor health and large disparities in health. Older adults, minorities, those from low SES backgrounds, and those who do not speak English as their primary language are the most affected.

Now the charge is to move forward with new solutions and ways to measure and test them. Health literacy has already come a long way since it was first conceived, and now plays a key role in widespread efforts to connect people to information and services that they can understand and use to improve their health. Health care providers are being trained to speak in simpler language and check for understanding; organizations are lowering barriers to care for people with literacy challenges; and all of these changes geared to adults with literacy challenges are making it easier for all of us, regardless of our literacy skills or educational backgrounds. In particular, they are helping all older adults to do things like talk with their doctors, manage their medicines, and find ways to stay active and healthy.

So where do we go from here? We build more momentum by creating new measures and testing different types of interventions; by creating an evidence base for best practices and knowing which practices work for different populations. We build momentum by breaking out of the confines of the exam room and the poorly written brochure, and learning more about how health literacy can be a tool that affects community and public health overall. We look at behavioral and social support and the reality of people's everyday lives. And finally, we build momentum by working on the positives. We know the problem well and now we can start to discover the best solutions.

As we mentioned at the beginning of the chapter, we encourage you to consider where do *you* want to go from here with health literacy? How will you contribute to improve health literacy and, in turn, health outcomes among older adults? We provided some potential direction and hope that you, as future gerontologists, incorporate your perspectives into the field of health literacy. We encourage your voices and look forward to where you go from here with health literacy!

REFERENCES

Auerbach, E. R. (1992). Making meaning, making change: Participatory curriculum development for adult ESL literacy. *Language in Education: Theory & Practice, 78*: ERIC.

Baker, D. W., Gazmararian, J. A., Sudano, J., & Patterson, M. (2000). The association between age and health literacy among elderly persons. *Journals of Gerontology: Series B: Psychological Sciences and Social Sciences, 55*(6), S368–S374.

Baker, D. W., Gazmararian, J. A., Williams, M. V., Scott, T., Parker, R. M., Green, D., . . . Peel, J. (2002). Functional health literacy and the risk of hospital admission among Medicare managed care enrollees. *American Journal of Public Health, 92*(8), 1278–1283.

Baldi, S., Kutner, M., Greenberg, E., Jin, Y., Baer, J., Moore, E., . . . White, S. (2009). *Technical report and data file user's manual for the 2003 National Assessment of Adult Literacy* (NCES 2009-476). U.S. Department of Education National Center for Education Statistics, Trans.

Brach, C., Keller, D., Hernandez, L. M., Baur, C., Parker, R., Dreyer, B., . . . Schillinger, D. (2012). *Ten attributes of health literate health care organizations.* Washington, DC: Institute of Medicine of the National Academies.

Coleman, C. A., Hudson, S., & Maine, L. L. (2013). Health literacy practices and educational competencies for health professionals: A consensus study. *Journal of Health Communication, 18*(Suppl. 1), 82–102.

Coleman, C., Kurtz-Rossi, S., McKinney, J., Pleasant, A., Rootman, I., & Shohet, L. (2009). *The Calgary charter on health literacy: Rationale and core principles for the development of health literacy curricula.* Calgary Institute on Health Literacy Curricula: The Centre for Literacy of Quebec.

Dowe, M. C., Lawrence, P. A., Carlson, J., & Keyserling, T. C. (1997). Patients' use of health-teaching materials at three readability levels. *Applied Nursing Research, 10*(2), 86–93.

Franklin, S. S., Thijs, L., Hansen, T. W., O'Brien, E., & Staessen, J. A. (2013). White-coat hypertension new insights from recent studies. *Hypertension, 62*(6), 982–987.

Freire, P. (1970). *Pedagogy of the oppressed*, translated by Myra Bergman Ramos. New York, NY: Continuum.

Haun, J. N., Valerio, M. A., McCormack, L. A., Sørensen, K., & Paasche-Orlow, M. K. (2014). Health Literacy Measurement: An inventory and descriptive summary of 51 instruments. *Journal of Health Communication, 19*(Suppl. 2), 302–333. doi:10.1080/10810730.2014.936571

Kirsch, I. S. (1993). *Adult literacy in America: A first look at the results of the National Adult Literacy Survey.* Washington, DC: United States Department of Education. ERIC (ED358375).

Knowles, M. (1973). *The adult learner: A neglected species.* Houston, TX: Gulf Publishing.

Knowles, M. (1992). *The modern practice of adult education: Andragogy versus pedagogy.* Author of the Classic Informal Adult Educator. New York, NY: Association Press.

Kutner, M., Greenburg, E., Jin, Y., & Paulsen, C. (2006). *The health literacy of America's adults: Results from the 2003 National Assessment of Adult Literacy.* Washington, DC: U.S. Department of Education.

McCormack, L., Bann, C., Squiers, L., Berkman, N. D., Squire, C., Schillinger, D., . . . Hibbard, J. (2010). Measuring health literacy: A pilot study of a new skills-based instrument. *Journal of Health Communication, 15*, 51–71.

Nielsen-Bohlman, L., Panzer, A., & Kindig, D. A. (2004). *Health literacy: A prescription to end confusion.* Washington, DC: National Academies Press.

Osborne, R. H., Batterham, R., Elsworth, G., Hawkins, M., & Buchbinder, R. (2013). The grounded psychometric development and initial validation of the Health Literacy Questionnaire (HLQ). *BioMed Central Public Health, 13*(1), 658.

Pearlin, L. I. (1989). The sociological study of stress. *Journal of Health and Social Behavior, 30*, 241–256.

Perls, T. T., Bochen, K., Freeman, M., Alpert, L., & Silver, M. H. (1999). Validity of reported age and centenarian prevalence in New England. *Age and Ageing, 28*(2), 193–197.

Pleasant, A. (2008). A second look at the health literacy of American adults and the National Assessment of Adult Literacy. *Focus on Basics, 46–52.*

Pleasant, A. (2014). Advancing health literacy measurement: A pathway to better health and health system performance. *Journal of Health Communication, 19*(12), 1481–1496. doi:10.1080/10810730.2014.954083

Pleasant, A., & McKinney, J. (2011). Coming to consensus on health literacy measurement: An online discussion and consensus-gauging process. *Nursing Outlook, 59*(2), 95–106.e101.

Pleasant, A., McKinney, J., & Rikard, R. V. (2011). Health literacy measurement: A proposed research agenda. *Journal of Health Communication, 16*(Suppl. 3), 11–21.

Ratzan, S. C., & Parker, R. M. (2000). Introduction. In C. R. Selden, M. Zorn, S. C. Ratzan, & R. M. Parker (Eds.), *National library of medicine current bibliographies in medicine: Health literacy.* NLM Pub. No. CBM 2000-1. Bethesda, MD: National Institutes of Health, U.S. Department of Health and Human Services.

Rootman, I., & Ronson, B. (2005). Literacy and health research in Canada: Where have we been and where should we go? *Canadiun Journal of Public Health, 96,* 562–577.

Rudd, R. E., Anderson, J. E., Oppenheimer, S., & Nath, C. (2007). Health literacy: An update of public health and medical literature. *Review of Adult Learning and Literacy, 7,* 175–204.

Sanders, L. M., Thompson, V. T., & Wilkinson, J. D. (2007). Caregiver health literacy and the use of child health services. *Pediatrics, 119*(1), e86–e92.

Smith, D., & Hudson, S. (2012). Using the person-environment-occupational-performance conceptual model as an analyzing framework for health literacy. *Journal of Communication in Healthcare, 5*(1), 3–11. doi:10.1179/175380761 1Y.0000000021

Sudore, R. L., Yaffe, K., Satter Field, S., Harris, T. B., Mehta, K. M., Simonsick, E. M., . . . Schillinger, D. (2006). Limited literacy and mortality in the elderly: The health, aging, and body composition study. *Journal of General Internal Medicine, 21*(8), 806–812.

Tsai, T. I., Lee, S. Y., Tsai, Y. W., & Kuo, K. (2011). Methodology and validation of health literacy scale development in Taiwan. *Journal of Health Communication, 16*(1), 50–61.

Williams, M. V., Baker, D. W., Parker, R. M., & Nurss, J. R. (1998). Relationship of functional health literacy to patients' knowledge of their chronic disease: A study of patients with hypertension and diabetes. *Archives of Internal Medicine, 158*(2), 166–172.

Index